MW01249300

HIV/AIDS

A Hazelden Pocket Health Guide

HIV/AIDS

*Practical, Medical, and Spiritual
Guidelines for Daily Living When
You're HIV-Positive*

MARK JENKINS

Foreword by Robert E. Larsen, M.D.

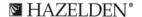

HAZELDEN®

INFORMATION & EDUCATIONAL SERVICES

Hazelden
Center City, Minnesota 55012-0176

1-800-328-0094
1-651-213-4590 (Fax)
www.hazelden.org

Library of Congress Cataloging-in-Publication Data
Jenkins, Mark, 1962–
    HIV/AIDS : practical, medical, and spiritual guidelines for daily living when
 you're HIV-positive / Mark Jenkins ; foreword by Robert E. Larsen.
       p. cm. — (A Hazelden pocket health guide)
    Includes bibliographical references and index.
    ISBN 1-56838-369-X
     1. AIDS (Disease)—Popular works. 2. AIDS (Disease)—Psychological aspects.
 I. Title. II. Series.

RC607.A26 J456 2000
616.97'92—dc21
                                                                    00-020074

04 03 02 01 00   6 5 4 3 2 1

Editor's note
The excerpt from the text *Alcoholics Anonymous,* pages 83–84, and the Twelve
Steps of Alcoholics Anonymous are reprinted and adapted with permission of
Alcoholics Anonymous World Services, Inc. (AAWS). Permission to reprint and
adapt the Twelve Steps does not mean that AAWS has reviewed or approved the
contents of this publication, or that AAWS necessarily agrees with the views ex-
pressed herein. AA is a program of recovery from alcoholism *only*—use of this excerpt and the Twelve Steps in connection with programs and activities which are
patterned after AA, but which address other problems, or in any other non-AA context, does not imply otherwise.

Cover design by David Spohn
Interior design by Donna Burch
Typesetting by Stanton Publication Services, Inc.

Contents

Foreword

For the past sixty years, millions of addicts and alcoholics have stopped using drugs and found new, rewarding lives by following the spiritual principles outlined in Twelve Step programs such as Alcoholics Anonymous. From a medical perspective, it is not unreasonable to say that Twelve Step programs constitute the gold standard of treatment for the chronic disease of chemical dependency. These programs have been so successful that they are now used to deal with other challenges of a chronic nature, such as overeating, sexual compulsion, gambling, and depression.

The Hazelden Pocket Health Guide series is designed to help patients cope with chronic diseases, specifically, diseases that may be the result of an addiction. These long-term, potentially debilitating illnesses include chronic obstructive pulmonary disease (COPD), hypertension, HIV/AIDS, and liver disease. This series can help patients use the same spiritual principles that have enabled so many chemically dependent people to lead full and satisfying lives.

Spirituality and acceptance are powerful tools patients and health care professionals can apply to help deal with disease. In thirty years of medical practice, I have seen many patients with chronic disease who, despite the best physicians and hospitals, have done poorly. Sometimes this was due to the severity of the disease process, but often, the patients' inability to accept the disease and its consequences was significant. Denial is a common problem in chemically dependent people, but chemical dependency is by no means the only disease in which it plays a major role in the outcome. Denial is common to *every* chronic disease known to medical science and if not dealt with effectively is a major stumbling block to effective treatment.

Despite significant advances in treating diabetes, for instance, at least half of all diabetics fail to follow their diets or to take their medications properly. Many of these patients suffer amputations, kidney failure and dialysis, heart attacks, and blindness partly due to their disease but mostly due to the denial that blinds them to effective treatment of the disease.

Denial and chronic disease can be dealt with by using spiritual principles. Spirituality is not religion, although some people achieve it in traditional religious communities. Spirituality is the concept that each of us has a Higher Power that can help us cope with life. For many this is the traditional God, while for others it may be nature, the recovering community, or a set of guiding principles. Each person has his or her own concept of a Higher Power. Spirituality is not a particular religious dogma but rather a concept that allows people to feel good about how they live their lives.

Bill Wilson, the cofounder of Alcoholics Anonymous, described spirituality as the concept that we can do together what we could not do alone. Spirituality is about community and being a part of a greater whole. Spirituality is we *not* me.

HIV/AIDS

For tens of thousands of people, however, these words will begin the difficult process of coping with a disease that remains uniformly fatal.

Dealing with the reality of being HIV-positive is one of the most difficult human experiences. The patient lives each day with uncertainty and fear and symptoms that at some point begin to accelerate in severity. Daily activities become more challenging as drug therapy and its side effects take on more of a presence in the patient's life. Rejection and fear from family and friends may lead to isolation and despair. How, then, is one to cope with such a situation?

Fortunately, the news about AIDS is not uniformly bad. Medical science has made significant inroads in treating this deadly disease. Patients are living longer and with less difficulty than ever before. Hope for treatments that will significantly increase life span is at its highest since the disease was discovered. For today's HIV-positive patient, the task is to live effectively while being treated and waiting for a breakthrough. The question is how to accomplish this task as well as is humanly possible.

Since the formation of Alcoholics Anonymous sixty years ago, people with an addictive disease have learned to live with a condition that is potentially fatal and that could recur at any time. Twelve Step programs, with their inherent spirituality, have been helping the HIV-positive patient to cope with the uncertainty of the future and the difficulty of the present. This Hazelden Pocket Health Guide is designed to help AIDS patients live to their fullest potential—physically, emotionally, and spiritually. Millions have been helped through the Twelve Steps. This book can help the HIV-positive patient cope with a very difficult disease.

Robert E. Larsen, M.D.
Coordinator, Health Care Professionals Program
Hazelden Foundation

Preface

I owe my life to a spiritual program of recovery. My journey started when I joined the recovery community. By following the Twelve Steps of Alcoholics Anonymous (the basis of *all* Twelve Step programs), I found a new life. My career was rebuilt; my relationships with others were mended; my self-esteem was restored.

A natural-born cynic, I was at first astounded when so many of "the Promises" I had been told about came true—and in such short order (see pages xxi–xxii for more on the Promises). By then I had learned not to question but to simply accept such blessings as part of my continuing journey in sobriety.

As a medical writer with several books to my credit, I began to postulate that this spiritual program of recovery from addiction would be a revelation to people living with chronic illnesses. After all, the Twelve Steps are a universal plan for living well. Countless groups apply the Twelve Steps to their addictions and conditions—everything ranging from Emotions Anonymous to Debtors Anonymous to Gamblers Anonymous to the grandparent of them all, Alcoholics Anonymous. And so I set about writing a book that offers a spiritual program of recovery from chronic illness.

Probably no one needs a guide to living well more than people who suffer from long-term medical conditions that dominate their lives. Chronic illness affects more than ninety million Americans and, according to the American Medical Association, is this nation's foremost health concern. Chronic illness leads to feelings of anger, isolation, and loneliness, financial difficulties, compromised personal relationships, and trouble at work. The emotional consequences of a chronic illness are especially profound when the condition is caused by a dependency on a mood-altering substance such as nicotine or alcohol. The Twelve Step program helps people deal with these overwhelming emotions by teaching them how to find their spirituality.

I am hardly the first person to suggest that the Twelve Steps can benefit those living with chronic illnesses. Many others whose lives have been transformed by a Twelve Step program have applied these principles to conditions ranging from cancer to AIDS.

However, what has been lacking in these interpretations is a plan for individual conditions. Until now.

This book is part of the Hazelden Pocket Health Guide series of books that adapts the Twelve Steps for those with chronic illnesses—in this case,

HIV/AIDS. The book combines specific medical guidelines with a plan to improve emotional and spiritual well-being. At its core is a program of hope, happiness, and healing.

Above all, this program provides those with chronic conditions and illnesses, such as HIV/AIDS, what they need: the indispensable tools and inspiration to live life one day at a time . . . and to *live it well*.

INTRODUCTION

Spirituality:
The Strongest Medicine of All?

Can spirituality help me beat my disease? That's probably the question you're asking yourself. A better question might be, Can the spiritual program this book teaches help me overcome the emotional pain of my disease so I can manage my disease more effectively? The answer to that question is "yes."

The National Institutes of Health recognizes spirituality as an important component of medical treatment. No wonder. A growing body of evidence suggests that spirituality actually helps people stay healthy and recover from illness.

In one of the most extensive laboratory studies ever done on the subject of spirituality and disease, researchers at Harvard's Mind/Body Medical Institute found that prayer and meditation—prerequisites for a sound spiritual life—cause a person's body to undergo healthful changes.[1] Metabolism, heart rate, and rate of breathing decrease, and brain waves slow down. These changes are the opposite of those induced by

1. For a brochure describing the Mind/Body Medical Institute, call (617) 632-9525 or visit its Web site at www.mindbody.harvard.edu

stress and are an effective therapy for certain diseases, especially those chronic in nature. Significantly, many doctors believe that because stress worsens a disease, a spiritual program that involves prayer and meditation is an effective component of treatment. If this is true, it is only logical to conclude that spirituality benefits those living with HIV/AIDS.

Although skeptics still question whether the chronically ill person who is spiritual is more likely to benefit medically than someone who is not spiritual, of this there is no doubt: spirituality helps chronically ill people cope with the emotional challenges of their condition.

But just what is spirituality anyway? One thing it *isn't* is religion. Although many truly religious people are spiritual, and many spiritual people consider themselves religious, the two concepts are not one and the same. A person doesn't have to be religious to be spiritual. Religion is a formalization of society's relationship with God into rituals and institutions. Spirituality is an inherent belief in the existence of a Higher Power, an energy, or a force—which a person may or may not choose to call God—and a feeling of closeness to that entity.

That being is referred to variously within these pages as a Higher Power, a Power greater than ourselves, or Power Greater.

This book advocates use of the Twelve Steps, a spiritual program founded in the 1930s to help alcoholics recover from the disease of alcoholism. The Twelve Steps can help you "turn over" care of your disease to a Higher Power that is greater and wiser than you and that loves you. The program will help you maintain strength and hope as you live each day with your disease.

You'll learn in depth about the Twelve Steps later in this book. Right now what's important is that you know that managing your HIV/AIDS[2] isn't just about addressing the medical aspects of the disease, although you will certainly learn most of what you need to know in these pages. No, managing HIV/AIDS is also about living well with that chronic illness every day.

The Twelve Steps will help you overcome your emotional pain by allowing you to recognize what you do and don't have control over. In cooperation with your Higher Power, you have the power to deal with your feelings about your disease and to change the behaviors that caused or exacerbated the condition, as well as to take certain steps to prevent it from getting worse, such as exercising, abstaining from alcohol,

2. The term *HIV/AIDS* is used throughout this book. It refers to people who are HIV-positive who may or may not yet have developed AIDS. Many of the recommendations in this book apply to people living with HIV whether or not they have developed AIDS, hence the use of this shorthand term.

and taking your medication. The Twelve Steps will also show you how to grow spiritually through prayer, meditation, and support.

Right now there is no cure for HIV/AIDS, just as there is no cure for alcoholism and other chronic illnesses. However, if you practice the principles outlined in the Twelve Steps, you will find the resolve you need to slow the progression of your HIV—and a way of life you may never have experienced had you not been stricken with a chronic illness.

Despite their popularity, Twelve Step programs are still widely misunderstood in some quarters. Such misunderstandings stand in the way of their acceptance by those who could really use them, including people with chronic illnesses such as HIV/AIDS. Perhaps the most common misunderstanding is that Twelve Step programs are "covers" for religion—specifically, Christian groups.

A hasty reading of the Steps may reinforce this impression. However, after reading more carefully, people soon discover that the Steps do not endorse any religion. A person who lives by the Steps could be Jewish, Christian, Hindu, Muslim, Buddhist, agnostic, or atheist.

If the Twelve Steps are not a religious program, then they certainly are a spiritual one. The Steps echo what writer Aldous Huxley called the "perennial philosophy"—a core set of ideas and practices shared by many religious traditions. The Steps have one major concern, and that is human transformation.

You may already be intimately familiar with a Twelve Step program. If you have not experienced the Steps, you will discover that they offer a new approach to living. This approach is available to you if you acknowledge your jeopardy and your need to change your behaviors and to improve your state of being.

The spiritual component of this book draws extensively on principles developed by the founders of Alcoholics Anonymous. Like alcoholism, HIV is a chronic disease. And as with alcoholics, if you don't do what's necessary to address your condition, your disease will come to profoundly affect your life.

Alcoholics must abstain from alcohol and other drugs. As a person living with HIV, you must follow a strict drug regimen and live a more healthy lifestyle. The extraordinary success achieved by millions of participants in Twelve Step programs who now abstain from alcohol and other drugs can be emulated by those with HIV/AIDS who follow the Steps suggested in this book.

It is heartening to know that the Promises that inspire Alcoholics Anonymous members also offer strength and hope to people with HIV/AIDS who are willing to follow this simple program:

If we are painstaking about this phase of our development, we will be amazed before we are half way through. We are going to know a new freedom and a new happiness. We will not regret the past nor wish to shut the door on it. We will comprehend the word serenity and we will know peace. No matter how far down the scale we have gone, we will see how our experience can benefit others. That feeling of uselessness and self-pity will disappear. We will lose interest in selfish things and gain interest in our fellows. Self-seeking will slip away. Our whole attitude and outlook upon life will change. Fear of people and of economic insecurity will leave us. We will intuitively know how to handle situations which used to baffle us. We will suddenly realize that God is doing for us what we could not do for ourselves.[3]

The Twelve Step program of spirituality discussed in this book stresses acceptance. Only when you accept that you have HIV and that it can cause serious health consequences will you be able to take the steps necessary to address the disease. Not only will denial prevent you from addressing the spiritual component of your chronic disease, but also in a very real way it will delay you from taking the vital medical measures

3. *Alcoholics Anonymous,* 3d ed. (New York: Alcoholics Anonymous World Services, Inc., 1976), 83–84. Reprinted with permission.

necessary to improve and extend your life. Thus the first part of this book describes HIV/AIDS, its symptoms and causes, and the basics of treatment.

The Twelve Steps for HIV/AIDS[4]

Step One—We admitted we were powerless over chronic illness—that our lives had become unmanageable.

Step Two—Came to believe that a Power greater than ourselves could restore us to sanity.

Step Three—Made a decision to turn our will and our lives over to the care of a Power greater than ourselves.

Step Four—Made a searching and fearless moral inventory of ourselves.

Step Five—Admitted to the God of our understanding, to ourselves, and to another human being the exact nature of our wrongs.

Step Six—Were entirely ready to have the God of our understanding remove all these defects of character.

Step Seven—Humbly asked our Higher Power to remove our shortcomings.

Step Eight—Made a list of all persons we had harmed, and became willing to make amends to them all.

---

4. Adapted from the Twelve Steps of Alcoholics Anonymous with the permission of AA World Services, Inc., New York, N.Y.

Step Nine—Made direct amends to such people wherever possible, except when to do so would injure them or others.

Step Ten—Continued to take personal inventory and when we were wrong promptly admitted it.

Step Eleven—Sought through prayer and meditation to improve our conscious contact with a Power greater than ourselves, praying only for knowledge of our Higher Power's will and the courage to carry that out.

Step Twelve—Having had a spiritual awakening as the result of these steps, we tried to carry our message to others with our condition and to practice these principles in all our affairs.

The Twelve Steps of Alcoholics Anonymous[5]

Step One—We admitted we were powerless over alcohol—that our lives had become unmanageable.

Step Two—Came to believe that a Power greater than ourselves could restore us to sanity.

Step Three—Made a decision to turn our will and our lives over to the care of God *as we understood Him.*

---

5. The Twelve Steps of AA are taken from *Alcoholics Anonymous,* 3d ed., published by AA World Services, Inc., New York, N.Y., 59–60. Reprinted with permission of AA World Services, Inc. (See editor's note on copyright page.)

Step Four—Made a searching and fearless moral inventory of ourselves.

Step Five—Admitted to God, to ourselves, and to another human being the exact nature of our wrongs.

Step Six—Were entirely ready to have God remove all these defects of character.

Step Seven—Humbly asked Him to remove our shortcomings.

Step Eight—Made a list of all persons we had harmed, and became willing to make amends to them all.

Step Nine—Made direct amends to such people wherever possible, except when to do so would injure them or others.

Step Ten—Continued to take personal inventory and when we were wrong promptly admitted it.

Step Eleven—Sought through prayer and meditation to improve our conscious contact with God *as we understood Him,* praying only for knowledge of His will for us and the power to carry that out.

Step Twelve—Having had a spiritual awakening as the result of these steps, we tried to carry this message to alcoholics, and to practice these principles in all our affairs.

CHAPTER ONE

The Essentials of HIV and AIDS

The AIDS pandemic is one of the most serious health crises in history. AIDS has resulted in the deaths of approximately 11.7 million people worldwide and will eventually cause the deaths of the estimated 33.4 million men, women, and children around the world now living with this disease. In 1998, roughly 6 million people were newly infected with HIV, the virus that causes AIDS—that's more than 16,000 people a day.

In North America, about 1 million people are HIV-positive. Each year, another 50,000 Americans become infected, including 2,500 infants. AIDS is now the leading cause of death for men between the ages of twenty-five and forty-four and the third-highest cause of death for women in the same age bracket.

Although there is no cure, people with HIV/AIDS are living longer, healthier, and more productive lives thanks to new and more effective treatments.

Early detection is key. Finding out early on whether you have HIV can help you in the following ways:

- You can get drug treatment—the sooner it starts, the more effective it will be.
- You can learn how to protect your health from further damage through diet and lifestyle changes.
- You can learn how to prevent transmitting the infection to others.
- You can tap into spiritual resources to help you cope with your disease.

This chapter will introduce you to the basics of HIV/AIDS and the fundamentals of its management. You might want to share this chapter or even the entire book with your friends and family. It will help them understand the challenges you face.

No single resource can be expected to address every issue. Always consult your doctor if you have any questions about your condition.

AIDS and HIV Explained

AIDS stands for *Acquired Immune Deficiency Syndrome*. Breaking the term down into its separate parts makes it easier to understand:

Acquired: You can catch it.

Immune Deficiency: A weakness in the body's mechanism to fight illness, known as the "immune system."

Syndrome: A group of symptoms that collectively indicate a disease.

Put simply, AIDS is a severe disorder of the immune system that makes you susceptible to common infections and diseases. These infections and diseases may kill you because your body's defense mechanism (the immune system) cannot fight them.

AIDS is caused by a virus called the *human immunodeficiency virus* (HIV). When HIV enters your body, it infects and kills your CD4+ cells. Sometimes called T-helper cells, CD4+ cells help your body fight infection and disease.

How Is HIV Transmitted?

HIV is transmitted from person to person through contact with body fluids that contain sufficient amounts of the virus. These body fluids include blood, vaginal fluid, semen (including pre-ejaculate, or "pre-cum"), and breast milk. It is possible to get HIV through oral sex, especially if you have open sores in your mouth or bleeding gums.

You can get HIV from anyone who is infected, even if the person doesn't appear sick and hasn't yet tested positive for HIV. The most common ways of contracting HIV are by having sex with an infected person; sharing needles when shooting drugs with an infected person; and being born to a woman who is infected or breast-feeding from a woman who is infected.

If you already have a sexually transmitted disease (STD), you are more likely to get infected with HIV. This is true when the STD in question causes open sores or breaks in the skin (e.g., syphilis, herpes, chancroid) and when it does not (e.g., chlamydia, gonorrhea). Also, when an HIV-infected person has another STD, that person is three to five times more likely than other HIV-infected people to transmit HIV through sexual activity.

Blood transfusions were at one time a common way people in the United States were infected with HIV. However, the national blood supply is now well screened and today infection via blood transfusion is almost unheard of.

You do not get HIV from

- donating blood
- bug bites (including mosquito bites)
- touching, hugging, or dry-kissing a person with HIV

- the urine or sweat of an infected person
- public restrooms, saunas, showers, or pools
- sharing towels or clothing
- sharing eating utensils or drinks
- socializing with a person who has HIV/AIDS

Why Injecting Drugs Can Cause HIV Infection

Every time an injection is given, blood from the person getting the injection enters the needle and syringe (the works). If a person who is HIV-positive is using the needle and syringe, then HIV-infected blood will contaminate the works. If the needle and syringe are shared with another person without being carefully cleaned—common behavior among some drug addicts—then HIV-infected blood gets injected straight into that person's bloodstream.

Sharing drug paraphernalia poses other risks for HIV transmission. The virus may be transmitted in blood in the following ways:

- *using blood-contaminated syringes when preparing drugs for use*
- *reusing water*
- *reusing bottle caps, spoons, or other containers to dissolve drugs in water and to heat drug solutions*

- *reusing small pieces of cotton or cigarette filters to filter out particles that could block the needle*

Street drug sellers often repackage used syringes and sell them as sterile. It is important to be aware that sharing a needle or syringe for any type of use, including skin popping and injecting steroids, can put you at risk for HIV and other blood-borne infections.

The Symptoms: How Do I Know If I Am HIV-Positive?

Initially, you may not be aware of having been infected with HIV. Some people develop flu-like symptoms such as fever, headache, sore muscles and joints, stomachache, swollen lymph glands, or a skin rash that lasts from one to two weeks. Many people have no symptoms at all.

However, over the course of weeks and months the virus begins to multiply. It will be some time before your immune system responds to the virus. Until that time, you will not test positive for HIV, though you can infect other people. Of course, this reinforces the importance of practicing safe sex and not sharing needles.

When your immune system responds—usually

after several months—it does so by producing antibodies in an attempt to destroy the virus. The test to detect HIV is actually a test to detect the presence of HIV antibodies. When your body eventually starts producing these antibodies, you will test positive for HIV.

After the initial symptoms—which may or may not be felt—some people with HIV remain healthy and symptom-free for ten years or more. But during this time the virus is attacking the immune system.

The most common way to measure the damage to your immune system is to count how many CD4+ cells you have. These cells are a crucial part of the immune system. A person with a healthy immune system has between 500 and 1,500 CD4+ cells per millimeter of blood.

As your CD4+ cell count drops, and your body is unable to fight the virus, you will probably start to experience unpleasant symptoms of HIV such as fevers, night sweats, diarrhea, or swollen lymph nodes. These symptoms will probably continue for several weeks.

When Does HIV Infection Become AIDS?

HIV disease becomes AIDS when your immune system is so damaged that you have fewer than 200 CD4+ cells or when you develop an *opportunistic infection*.

The U.S. government's Centers for Disease Control (CDC) puts out an official list of opportunistic infections. According to the CDC, a person with HIV who develops one of these conditions is defined as having AIDS, whether or not his or her CD4+ cell count is below 200. Some of the most common opportunistic infections are as follows:

- Pneumocystis carinii pneumonia (PCP), a lung infection
- Kaposi's sarcoma (KS), a skin cancer
- cytomegalovirus (CMV), an infection that usually affects the eyes
- candida, a fungus that can cause thrush (a white film in your mouth) or infections in your throat or vagina

AIDS also causes severe weight loss, brain tumors, and other serious health problems that, unless treated, can be fatal.

AIDS affects every infected person differently. Some people die within a year of getting infected, while others live for many years, even after being diagnosed with AIDS.

Getting Tested

If you think you may have been exposed to HIV, it is extremely important to get tested. If you have HIV, the sooner you start treatment for the virus, the more effective treatment will be, and you will get a head start on measures to protect your overall health. Also, if you know you have AIDS, you will need to learn to protect others from catching the virus from you.

Thinking about getting tested can provoke intense anxiety. Frequently, people avoid getting tested because they are afraid of testing positive. Think about the situation this way: if you *do* have HIV, you are going to find out sometime; if you find out early, you will have an opportunity to slow the progression of the disease and to prevent or lessen many of the signs and symptoms of HIV/AIDS.

You should definitely be tested for HIV if you answer yes to one or more of the following questions:

- Did you have a blood transfusion before 1985?
- Have you ever injected drugs into your body?
- Are you a health care worker?
- Have you had a tattoo done on your body or had any part of your body pierced?
- Have you had multiple sex partners?
- Does your partner have HIV or AIDS?
- Is your partner in a high-risk group for HIV or AIDS?

Many places offer testing for HIV infection, including your local health department, offices of private doctors, hospitals, and, of course, sites specifically established to provide HIV testing.

It is important to be tested someplace that also provides HIV/AIDS counseling. Counselors will answer your questions about high-risk behaviors and ways to protect yourself and others in the future. Also, they can help you interpret the test results and describe HIV/AIDS-related resources available where you live.

If you have questions about testing or want to find a testing site in your area, call the Centers for Disease Control National AIDS Hotline at (800) 342-2437.

The standard test to detect HIV is a blood test called *enzyme immunoassay* (EIA). This test looks for antibodies your body produces to fight the virus. If the diagnosis is positive, the result will be confirmed with another test, such as a Western blot, before being given to you.

Rapid Tests

It may take from one to two weeks to get the result of an EIA. It takes between five and thirty minutes to get results from so-called rapid tests. The only rapid test currently licensed by the Food and Drug Administration (FDA) for use in the United States is the Single Use Diagnostic System (SUDS). The availability of rapid tests will vary depending on where you live. The rapid HIV test is as accurate as the EIA. As with the EIA, rapid tests must be used with a confirmatory test, such as the Western blot, before a diagnosis of infection can be given.

Other Tests

Tests other than the EIA and rapid tests are available to detect HIV. These tests are generally expensive because they require sophisticated equipment and special training. They are rarely used to test individuals; instead, they are used to test the blood supply and for research purposes.

When Should You Get Tested?

Most HIV tests look for antibodies produced by your body to fight the virus. The majority of people develop measurable amounts of these antibodies within three months of being infected (the average is twenty-five days). In rare cases, it can take six months. Thus you should get tested six months after the last possible exposure (unprotected vaginal, anal, or oral sex or sharing needles). It is highly unlikely that it would take longer than six months for a person to develop detectable antibodies. Because you may not test positive until six months after infection, it is extremely important you protect yourself and others from further exposure to HIV.

What Does Your Test Result Reveal about Your Sex Partner?

Many people wonder, If my HIV test shows I don't have the virus, does that mean my sex partner is HIV-negative too? The answer is no! HIV is not necessarily transmitted every time you have sex. In other words, your sex partner may have HIV, but hasn't transmitted it to you—*yet*. Testing should never take the place of protecting yourself from being infected with HIV. If your behavior is putting you at risk, change your behavior. And, of course, encourage your sex partner to get tested. Until the result comes back, the two of you should practice safe sex.

Pregnancy and Testing

Pregnant women should get tested for HIV. Drug therapies can now lower the chance that an HIV-infected expectant mother will pass on HIV to her infant before, during, or after birth. The drug used to reduce perinatal transmission is zidovudine (ZDV), also known as AZT or Retrovir. HIV testing and counseling give pregnant women who are infected with HIV the opportunity to gain access to medical treatment that may help delay disease transmission. For women who are not infected, the counseling available with testing provides the chance to learn important ways to avoid getting HIV.

What If I Test Positive for HIV?

As soon as possible, see a doctor who specializes in treating HIV and AIDS. Many drugs are now available to treat HIV and help you maintain good health. You should start thinking immediately about such treatments.

Testing for HIV at Home

Home-test HIV kits are available. Several types are advertised for sale, although the FDA has approved only one such product called Home Access. The accuracy of other products is unverified.

Home Access is sold in most drugstores. To use the kit, you prick your finger with a special implement and place the drops of blood on a specially treated card. Then you mail the card to a licensed facility to be tested. To ensure confidentiality, clients are provided an identification number to use when calling for the result. Callers may speak with a counselor before taking the test, while waiting for the test result, and when getting the result.

How to Protect Others When You Have HIV:

- *Never have unprotected sex. Unprotected sex is sex without a condom. Not having sex (abstinence) is the best way to protect others. If you are sexually active, use a new latex condom every time.*

- *If you use a lubricant, make sure it is water-based. Do not use petroleum-based lubricants, cold cream, baby oil, or other oils because they can make the condom break.*

- *If you are allergic to latex, use polyurethane condoms.*

- *If no male condoms are available, use female condoms.*

- *If you choose to use a spermicide (a cream, foam, or gel for killing sperm), do as the instructions say. You can use condoms with or without spermicide.*

- *For oral sex, use protection such as a condom, dental dam (a square piece of latex used by dentists), or plastic food wrap. Do not reuse these items.*

- *Keep sex toys for your own use only and don't use anyone else's sex toys.*

- *Don't share drug needles or drug works. If you are a drug addict, seek help for your addiction (see pages 60–61).*

- *Inform current and former sex partners that you have HIV. This can be difficult, but it is important so they can get the help they need if you have transmitted the virus to them.*

*Your local public health department may
help you find these people.*

- *If a woman you had sex with is pregnant,
even if you are not the father, it is very important that you tell her you have HIV. If she
has HIV, she needs to get early medical care
for her own health and that of her baby.*

- *Don't donate blood, plasma, or organs.*

- *Keep personal care items such as razors and
toothbrushes for your own use only and don't
use someone else's—HIV can be transmitted
through fresh blood on such items.*

Is There a Cure for AIDS?

At present there is no cure for AIDS. Medicines can
slow the progression of HIV and slow the damage the
virus does to your immune system. There is no way,
however, to get all the HIV out of your body. AIDS
researchers hope that the new, more powerful anti-
HIV drugs might eventually kill off the virus if they
are taken for several years, but there is no evidence
this is happening.

You can take other medications to prevent or treat
some of the opportunistic infections. Some diseases
respond well to such treatments, while others do not.
And certain people respond better than others to particular drug treatments.

Once a diagnosis is made, the most important goal is to begin an appropriate treatment program. These are the components of a successful program to manage HIV and AIDS:

- Get the right medical treatment for your condition (chapter 3).
- Participate in a Twelve Step program of spirituality (chapter 2).
- Learn to live on a daily basis with your symptoms (chapter 4).

Where to Get Government-Approved Information about HIV Treatments

If you test positive for HIV, seek the care of a doctor or medical service with experience in treating people with HIV and AIDS—and, ideally, one who specializes in this area of medicine.

In-depth information on specific treatments is also available from the HIV/AIDS Treatment Information Service (ATIS) by calling (800) 448-0440.

Information on participating in clinical trials is available from the AIDS Clinical Trials Information Service (ACTIS) by calling (800) 874-2572 or logging on to www.actis.org.

The Centers for Disease Control National

AIDS Hotline offers practical information about a variety of treatments. You can reach it at (800) 342-2437. The hotline can also provide referrals to national treatment hotlines, local AIDS organizations, and health care providers experienced in HIV and AIDS management.

The Mind-Body Connection

Strong evidence suggests that spirituality is a fundamental component of extending survival rates for chronic illness. In addition to the physical benefits of prayer and meditation, which have been properly documented, practicing the principles of a spiritual program enhances a person's ability to cope emotionally with chronic conditions such as HIV and AIDS.

Such coping skills are greatly needed. Because there are often no symptoms early on, or the symptoms are very mild, people diagnosed with HIV may have difficulty accepting either that they have the disease or that it has serious consequences for them. As a result, they may not take the necessary measures to address it. Acceptance is an integral component of an effective spiritual program for chronic illness. If and when a person does accept the diagnosis, emotions such as anger, frustration, anxiety, and depression are apt to surface. A spiritual program for chronic illness can help alleviate such feelings.

Psychological Impact of HIV/AIDS

The psychological impact of a chronic illness such as HIV/AIDS can be as devastating as the physical symptoms. The following psychological symptoms, which may occur quite apart from the symptoms of the disease itself, are commonly associated with HIV/AIDS:

- *profound, persistent episodes of sadness lasting for longer than two weeks*
- *loss of interest in favorite activities*
- *difficulty sleeping*
- *feeling depressed most of the day*
- *decreased sexual drive*
- *feelings of worthlessness*
- *difficulty concentrating*
- *absentmindedness*
- *recurrent thoughts of suicide*

These are all signs and symptoms of depression, which is common in patients with chronic diseases. The presence of depression reinforces the need for health care for HIV/AIDS patients that goes beyond medical treatment. Doctors recommend that people with these symptoms seek help from a mental health professional, such as a therapist, and join a support group where members share common experiences and problems.

CHAPTER TWO

A Spiritual Program
to Help Manage HIV/AIDS

Living with HIV/AIDS may be the biggest challenge you ever face. You will probably have to undergo bouts of drug therapy, which can be overwhelming. It can be all the more trying if the therapy doesn't appear to be working. For a disease that may not show any symptoms, you could endure disruptive yet necessary drug therapy that has major side effects.

Developing the resolve to manage your HIV/AIDS will require making changes, not just to your daily routine but to the way you look at life. Making these changes can provide you with the opportunity to live a life that is more happy, joyous, and free—a life that may be better than you've ever known.

The question is, How do you go about this?

To achieve the resolve to successfully address your disease, you need a spiritual plan as well as a medical one. The Twelve Step program referred to throughout this book is such a spiritual program. It has worked with astonishing success for millions of people with the chronic illnesses of addiction, including alcoholism and other drug addictions, gambling, and overeating. Its principles have provided great comfort and relief for people with other chronic illnesses as well.

The Twelve Step program is, at its core, spiritual. It is strictly nondenominational, however, and accommodates people of all faiths. The program also welcomes those who do not have religious faith. Nevertheless, success in this program requires a profound change in thinking from self-centeredness to acceptance of a "Higher Power" beyond oneself.

Twelve Step How-To

Thanks to the foresight of those who created the Twelve Step program, this guide to better living with chronic illness is flexible. This set of principles makes no draconian demands on you but rather offers suggestions for behavior that will result in an improved life with less emotional pain and greater spiritual living.

There is no rule about how the Steps should be done; this is a matter of personal preference. Many people with chronic illnesses have experienced great improvement in their spiritual well-being by doing the Steps selectively. However, the Twelve Steps build on each other. People who have followed them in sequence have found they work best that way. If you get a firm foothold on one Step before you go on to the next, you journey from acceptance to serenity one Step at a time.

Many people ask if there is a time frame for doing the Steps. "As long as it takes" is probably the best advice. But it is important to feel you are making progress. As far as possible, don't become stalled on one Step or take lengthy breaks between them.

And keep in mind that doing the Steps isn't a one-time thing. You continue to practice the principles of the Steps in your daily life, and there is nothing to stop you from starting again on Step One and working all the way to Step Twelve whenever you wish. For many people, "working the Steps" provides tremendous serenity and satisfaction, not to mention a simple plan for living well.

A careful reading of this part of the book will reveal that the underlying concepts of the Twelve Steps are not unique. Those who developed the Twelve Steps simply reflected on how they got sober. But their experience is supported by the collective sagacity of philosophers and religious leaders from different cultures throughout the ages. You will soon see that the message in the Steps is ageless; the philosophy is timeless; and the strength and hope offered to those with chronic illnesses such as HIV/AIDS are everlasting.

Much has been written about the Twelve Steps. The following pages will introduce you to each Step. If this is your first encounter with the Steps, you may find it helpful to gather more information. If you've been exposed to the Steps or currently work the program for an addiction, this chapter can serve as a review.

Step One: The Foundation of Recovery

We admitted we were powerless over chronic illness—that our lives had become unmanageable.

We've probably all heard it said that the first step is the hardest to take. This is certainly true with the Twelve Steps. In taking Step One, we must admit that we have HIV and that a very important part of our lives—our health—is out of control. Who wants to do such a thing?

Step One gets us to face reality. We cannot alter the fact that we have a virus in our bodies that wants to kill us. This is something we must accept. We are powerless to change that fact.

If we have become consumed by the knowledge that we have a chronic disease—and are experiencing depression, anger, fear, and anxiety—then our lives have become unmanageable.

The First Step takes courage. We have to admit

things about ourselves that we would prefer not to. Many of us with HIV/AIDS have to see that our disease is a consequence of choices we made in the past. Some of us have to deal with the anger that results from knowing we contracted the disease through no fault of our own. Like thousands who have gone before us, we can summon the courage to take this Step, the first in our spiritual journey toward achieving the serenity to manage our disease in its entirety.

Step Two: A Promise of Hope

Came to believe that a Power greater than ourselves could restore us to sanity.

Spirituality is an integral part of any Twelve Step program for chronic illness. Why? Because finding the serenity and strength to manage HIV/AIDS requires turning to a Power beyond ourselves.

Many of us already believe in a Higher Power we call God. If we don't believe in a Power greater than ourselves, it's important we at least stay open-minded about the concept. Even the slightest amount of faith that a Higher Power can and will help us is better than no faith at all. If this proves difficult, we "act as if" we believe, so we're open to experiencing its power.

Indeed, Step Two does not mean we must come to believe in God as presented in a formal religious context. If we think this is the case, we might dismiss the Twelve Step program because we think it won't work for us. Or, if we are religious, we may view the Steps as some sort of cult. We need to keep an open mind. Like all the Steps, Step Two is a suggestion from others who say, "This is the way it worked for us." Such people have found that the Second Step gave them hope—and there is hope for us if we come to believe that the source of power we need lies outside ourselves.

If we were to ask people with HIV/AIDS who have been restored to sanity how they identify their Higher Power, we would probably hear answers as varied as humankind's ideas on faith. Some might say God as they understand Him from the faith of their upbringing (the Christian God, for example); others might say God working through the Twelve Step program; and others might say their Power Greater was the Twelve Steps themselves, along with support group attendance and fellowship. They would undoubtedly tell us that their relationship with their Higher Power helped them step outside themselves and realize they are not the center of the universe.

On Insanity

"Restore me to sanity? But I'm not insane!" That might be your response to the second part of Step Two. Insanity here refers to our tendency to steadfastly refuse to acknowledge our

HIV/AIDS—even after we've been told that unless we do something, we'll suffer deadly consequences. The *American Heritage Dictionary* defines *insane* as being foolish or absurd. Most people would agree that not taking the clear-cut measures necessary to control a life-threatening disease meets the definition of foolish or absurd.

Step Three: Turning It Over

Made a decision to turn our will and our lives over to the care of a Power greater than ourselves.

Of all the Steps, the Third Step can be the most effective in helping us transcend the emotional pain of chronic illness. Time and time again, Step Three has provided what people needed to get through difficult moments and helped them approach the management of their disease with remarkable resolve.

In Step One we admitted we were powerless over the fact that we have HIV/AIDS and that our disease has made our lives unmanageable. In Step Two we came to believe that a Higher Power could help us get through our emotional pain. In Step Three we make the decision to let our Higher Power relieve us from the emotional pain and unmanageability of our disease and show us what we can do ourselves.

Turning our will over to a Power greater than

ourselves doesn't absolve us from doing whatever is necessary to care for ourselves. Our Higher Power loves us whatever we do and helps us by showing us how to help ourselves. Our Higher Power speaks through others and through us. We learn to listen to our feelings and to act on them.

No longer will we try to force impossible solutions or beliefs that aren't in our best interest. We won't expend time and energy "willing" our disease to go away. We let our Higher Power determine the best way for us to handle our disease and all the emotions that go along with it.

It is the responsibility of each and every one of us with HIV/AIDS to cooperate with our Higher Power. We need to do all we can to improve ourselves physically, mentally, spiritually, and emotionally.

Turning our will and our lives over to the care of a Higher Power doesn't "cure" our HIV/AIDS. But it does help us handle the challenge of managing our disease. It gives us the ability to consider a plan or purpose higher than our own.

Achieving the balance between letting our Higher Power care for us and taking personal responsibility can be hard. We discover how to achieve this balance by communicating with our Higher Power through prayer and meditation. In this way the answers are often revealed.

Once we have begun the process of "turning it over," we begin to find the resolve to manage our HIV/AIDS. We can halt, go inside ourselves, and in the tranquillity simply say the Serenity Prayer: "God, grant me the serenity to accept the things I cannot change, the courage to change the things I can, and the wisdom to know the difference. Thy will, not mine, be done."

Step Four: Knowing Yourself

Made a searching and fearless moral inventory of ourselves.

The importance of doing an inventory is to know ourselves better. By being searching and fearless about our liabilities, we gain insight into how we may have developed HIV/AIDS and why we react the way we do. Writing down an inventory helps us to understand what we need to do to correct the behaviors that may have brought us to this point and which ways of living will best help us manage our disease.

In doing this Step, we must be *moral* but not *moralistic*. Our behavior has been good and bad—that is the reality. We must examine it. Make it ours. Many of us contracted HIV/AIDS through no fault of our own—perhaps during a blood transfusion, though today this is unheard of. But some of us developed the virus as a result of destructive behaviors, such as

intravenous drug use or unsafe sex with multiple partners. We also need to examine our behavior since
being diagnosed with HIV/AIDS. We may have been
refusing to acknowledge that our falling CD4+ cell
count means we're "really" sick—after all, we don't
have any symptoms. And what about the impact emotionally? Have we indulged in excessive self-pity and
ignored our doctors' recommendations? Have we
taken out our frustrations and displeasure on our family members and friends? Do we continue to use intravenous drugs or engage in unprotected sex?

In doing our inventories, we shouldn't restrict ourselves to listing behavior having only to do with our
HIV/AIDS. It is important for us that we recognize
flaws that may have nothing to do with whether we
contracted the virus.

We must not punish ourselves for these behaviors.
The goal is to know ourselves and to accept ourselves.
Only when we see ourselves in a way that is enlight-
ening, not judgmental, can we strive to do better.

There are several ways to go about Step Four.
The most common way is to use a straightforward,
double-column list of specific positive and negative
behaviors.

Keep in mind that Step Four is not a test; we cannot fail it.

Taking the Fourth Step is a profound yet simple

start to an ongoing way of daily living. It is the beginning of a path to self-awareness, a way to go today and each day hereafter. The inventory becomes a way of life based on the courage and willingness to be completely honest to oneself about oneself.

This self-assessment may be the most difficult feat of our lives. If we need encouragement, support, or help, we can ask for it from someone we trust, such as a chaplain or counselor—someone who will be nonjudgmental.

When we have completed our Fourth Step inventories, we will possess more self-awareness and self-acceptance. We're now ready for the Fifth Step. We're now ready to make some changes in our lives and in the ways we manage our disease.

Step Five: Telling My Story

Admitted to the God of our understanding, to ourselves, and to another human being the exact nature of our wrongs.

In the Fifth Step we openly, honestly, and willingly share who we are. This is a time for introspection as well as for laying ourselves bare. It allows us to let our Higher Power and another person see us for who we really are—flawed but lovable people who really *are* capable of taking the measures necessary to manage our HIV/AIDS.

Step Five gives us the chance to rid ourselves of the hidden side of ourselves, the side that sometimes causes us to feel shame.

We need to prepare for this Step. True self-awareness and honesty do not come easily to most people. We are used to avoiding our character defects. To stand and actually face ourselves as we truly are is a difficult and spiritually demanding proposition.

The key to a good Step Five is to have done a thorough, balanced, and honest Fourth Step. In particular, the rigorous self-honesty called for in Step Four helps us to gain the *humility* we need to do an effective Step Five.

To Admit to a Higher Power

With the help of a Higher Power, we can find the inner courage and strength we need to take the Fifth Step. Caring, loving, and forgiving, our Higher Power will help us realize that we are not the only ones who fall short.

To Admit to Ourselves

To admit to ourselves where we went wrong is a sign that we are practicing true self-honesty. But it isn't easy. Who wants to confess to character flaws that may have caused a chronic illness? We go through our lives ignoring the ways we inflicted damage on our own bodies. Really, though, we do not forget. The knowledge gnaws inside us.

Taking the Fifth Step without being totally self-honest is self-defeating and merely perpetuates our negative feelings toward ourselves.

To do this Step well, it is important to love and respect ourselves. Step Five allows us to reflect on whether we are coping with our disease in a loving and nonjudgmental way. It gives us the chance to accept ourselves as flawed human beings. It lets us understand that we need forgiveness and another chance at life. When we forgive ourselves, we become free from the grip of guilt and shame.

To admit first to ourselves before admitting to another person shows we are willing to be really honest. We prove we are not afraid to face our real selves squarely. True honesty begins with this kind of self-honesty. Knowing ourselves and our strengths and weaknesses intimately can profoundly help us overcome any perceived obstacles to managing our HIV/AIDS.

To Admit to Another Person

We share the Fifth Step with another person. Why? Because sharing with another person the exact nature of our wrongs keeps us honest. By doing this Step, we allow another person to see us as complete, but flawed, human beings. Most of us will find this to be the hardest part of the Fifth Step. We may experience an overwhelming fear of embarrassment. But there is a great amount of relief in doing this. We no longer have to put energy into making others believe we're perfect.

Step Five is the opportunity to "cast out" those behaviors and traits that cause us emotional pain. It is not enough to acknowledge the nature of our wrongs to ourselves and through prayer to a Higher Power. It is only by speaking out—admitting out loud our mistakes, failures, and anxieties to another person—that the feelings and deeds lose their power over us. For those of us with a chronic illness such as HIV/AIDS, the Fifth Step is one major step away from a sense of isolation and loneliness; it is a step toward wholeness, happiness, and a real sense of gratitude.

Which "Human Being"?

During Step Five, most people wonder with whom they should share their secrets. The fact is that almost anyone will do—a clergy person, a doctor, a psychologist, a family member who won't be adversely affected by your total honesty, a counselor, a friend, or even a stranger. The best candidates have the following qualities:

- *discretion*
- *maturity and wisdom*
- *willingness to share their own experiences*
- *familiarity with the challenges of a chronic illness*

Often, such people are not readily available to us. One of our responsibilities in doing the Fifth Step is to look around carefully for someone who meets these criteria.

Whomever we decide to share our Fifth Step with, remember our intention is not to please that person but to heal ourselves. It is our inner selves we are trying to satisfy. We should also not be afraid of shocking listeners with our revelations.

Steps Four and Five Are Ongoing

The "housecleaning" process we do in Steps Four and Five is not meant to be a onetime event. As we will learn in Step Ten, regular personal inventories are measures we can take to help us transcend the emotional pain of our chronic disease and better manage our condition. If and when we decide to do these Steps again, we do not need to go back over our whole lives unless we continue to carry anger or other unresolved feelings or realize we overlooked a behavior we would like to change. Otherwise, we pick up where we left off when we last took inventory. What is past is past. Whenever we take another Fourth and Fifth Step, it can become an opportunity for increased self-knowledge, self-acceptance, and learning to forgive and seek forgiveness as a way of daily living.

Step Six: Ready, Willing, and Able

Were entirely ready to have the God of our understanding remove all these defects of character.

In Step One we admitted we were powerless over the fact that we now have HIV/AIDS. In Step Two we came to believe that a Higher Power could help us. In Step Three we made the decision to let that Power care for our lives. Steps Four and Five uncovered our defects of character.

If we have done these first five Steps honestly and thoroughly, we will be ready to let go of our character defects. The *readiness* to have them removed is the key to the Sixth Step. By being willing to let go of these character defects, we increase our chances of coping with our chronic illness.

In taking Step Six, we need to revisit that concept of powerlessness. Instead of telling our Higher Power what it is we want to be—"Make me more motivated" or "Make me more open-minded"—we make a statement of our condition as it is. We state how things are with us: "My Higher Power, I am lazy" or "My Higher Power, I am intolerant of others." Only with this humility will we be ready and willing to have such defects removed.

Even with all the preparation we do for the Sixth Step, we may still have reservations. Even when we know we no longer have any use for our defects of character, we've grown accustomed to them over the years. In our minds, our pride and selfishness served us well. We might ask ourselves, Can I let go of some of my most monumental defects?

That is why we go to the Seventh Step. It's there that we see our Higher Power doing for us what we really could not do for ourselves. For many, the removal of our shortcomings is the miracle that turns doubters into believers. Step Six is really the "get ready, get set" that builds toward the "go" of Step Seven—the *action* of asking our Higher Power to remove our shortcomings.

Step Seven: Being Changed

Humbly asked our Higher Power to remove our shortcomings.

The first word in Step Seven is *humbly*. Because Step Seven so expressly concerns itself with humility, we need to stop to consider its importance.

Humility is the practice of being humble. It is the recognition of our self-worth and seeing that same God-given worth in other people, even when they are so totally unlike us that we don't understand them or get along with them. Humility is the awareness that we are *not* all-powerful controllers of every aspect of our lives and that we do need the help and guidance of a Higher Power.

"Humbly" asking our Higher Power is quite different from the way we may be used to praying—either begging or bargaining. In those cases, we prayed to our Higher Power out of desperation. From now on we pray with humility; we humbly ask our Higher Power to remove our shortcomings.

Most people find it easier to ask that their shortcomings be removed gradually or one at a time. Having lived with these shortcomings for so long, we find it difficult to shed them all at once. We need to be patient with ourselves and with our Higher Power during this process. This may take time, a lot of work on our part, and more of the being "entirely ready" of Step Six. We don't expect to become perfect people, but we aim to improve. The goal is progress, not perfection.

We can work this Step alone with our Higher Power, with members of a religious group, or in support groups (for alcoholism, narcotics addiction, or HIV/AIDS, for instance)—wherever we can trust and be trusted.

And although a personal prayer is our own connection with our Higher Power, when two or three are gathered together, we feel a special bond not only with our Higher Power but also with others who share our condition. We feel this closeness as we say the Serenity Prayer together in our groups.

Our own shortcomings *can,* with our Higher Power's help, be removed.

Step Eight: Preparing for Change

Made a list of all persons we had harmed, and became willing to make amends to them all.

Step Eight adds even more strength to our program. If we have harmed others, it is important to make a heartfelt attempt to reconcile with them and to release our guilt. If we have hurt friends and the friendships have suffered, the benefit is that we might repair those friendships. By making a list, we become clear as to exactly who these people are.

Over the years, some of our behaviors, such as drug use or promiscuity, may have caused discomfort to others—to family, friends, and co-workers. We may have been rude to them when they asked us to stop a particular behavior. Chances are that at the very least we ignored or rebuffed many people's feelings on the subject.

We might want to consider what our behavior was like after we found out we had HIV/AIDS. It may have been unacceptable. We may have been disrespectful at times to the health care professionals who were trying to help us with our treatment. Our list needs to include all persons we've harmed, regardless of how much and under what circumstances.

We may want to put ourselves at the top of our amends list. We are the ones whose health may be suffering as a result of our actions.

Understandably, the prospect of acknowledging our responsibility for hurting others can be daunting. As with the other Steps, Step Eight becomes less frightening once we settle down to do it.

We can take some time to write the names of a few people who make us feel uncomfortable. We don't need to write why or anything else. This simple act of writing down names changes our perspective. Instead of thinking about the harm others have done to us, we take responsibility for the pain we caused in those relationships. It is a profound experience that represents a coming of age.

If you made a list, congratulations. You are halfway through this important Step.

Many of us avoid the Eighth Step because we are already thinking ahead to Step Nine or because we feel too guilty or fearful to face a long list of names. It is important to remember that just because we've written a list does not mean we need to make amends immediately.

The second part of this Step involves willingness. Being willing to make amends means discarding all resentments and accepting responsibility for the harm we have done to others.

In so doing we become completely ready to do whatever we can to make amends for these harms, thereby unburdening ourselves of guilty feelings that interfere with our emotional well-being as we contend with our HIV/AIDS.

Continuing to Make Amends

The Twelve Step program is not a program of perfection. Instead, it stresses progress. Even when we practice the principles of the program in all our affairs, it is inevitable we will have "run-ins" with other people in our lives (though far fewer than before, it is hoped). For that reason a new and revised Step Eight list is an option for any of us at any time.

Step Nine: Repairing the Past

Made direct amends to such people wherever possible, except when to do so would injure them or others.

We begin making amends to our loved ones by showing them we are caring for ourselves. In addition to protecting our bodies against substances that might be harmful—and in general treating our bodies better—we follow our doctors' recommendations for drug therapy and submit to follow-up therapy when necessary. No longer do our families and friends have to fear we are, through inaction, killing ourselves. We make many of our amends by taking appropriate measures to contain our disease.

These, though, are "indirect" amends, and the operative word in Step Nine is *direct*. Making amends directly helps us gain humility, honesty, and courage. That means we need to go to the people we have harmed and admit our wrongs. Being direct isn't just about righting wrongs. It also inspires us to summon honesty and courage to our service and gives us the freedom to look others in the eye and experience the self-respect we deserve.

An amend need not consist of a lengthy explanation. All that's needed is a heartfelt apology. The person to whom we are making the amend may feel some uneasiness too. For this reason, simplicity and directness usually work best when making the amend.

Ideally we apologize face-to-face. The very directness of this approach is beneficial. Sometimes this is impractical, however, so we may choose to write a letter, make a phone call, or even, in this electronic age, send an e-mail.

In the vast majority of cases, amends are well received. Even in those rare instances when they are not, this is not a reason to avoid the effort the next time. Almost always, relationships improve markedly when amends are made.

Steps Eight and Nine also allow us to make amends to *ourselves*. The reward for taking these Steps is a gradual but increasing sense of self-acceptance and self-respect, of being in harmony with our own personal world. Such feelings are indispensable in our quest to cope better with the challenges of our chronic illness.

Step Ten: Maintaining Your New Life

Continued to take personal inventory and when we were wrong promptly admitted it.

Managing our chronic illness presents us with a tremendous challenge. Yet by following the Steps of this program, we have been able to achieve a strong measure of conciliation with ourselves, others, and a Higher Power. To help maintain our serenity, we must try to stay comfortable with ourselves and others. We do this by continuing to take a personal inventory.

We are only human. The path we are taking offers progress, not perfection, so it is inevitable—even with a Higher Power in our lives—that we will do things that we know are wrong or misguided. These can be monumental or trivial. Maybe we have let our condition deteriorate, and the distressing symptoms caused us to entertain thoughts of suicide. Or the expense of a medication caused us to snap angrily at a pharmacist. When defects such as self-pity and anger rear up, we can go back and do a Seventh Step on them, asking our Higher Power to remove these shortcomings.

It helps to get feedback from people close to us— family, friends, fellow members of support groups. We need to ask these people to point out our character defects to us if they become apparent.

The second part of this Step emphasizes that if we want to maintain our serenity, we must admit our wrongs "promptly." It is important not to let anything build up inside us that will interfere with our ability to cope with our chronic illness. Once we get used to it, admitting we were wrong can be a liberating sensation that enables us to move on in our lives without harboring resentments or other unhealthy thoughts.

Step Eleven: Partnership with a Higher Power

Sought through prayer and meditation to improve our conscious contact with a Power greater than ourselves, praying only for knowledge of our Higher Power's will and the courage to carry that out.

When coping with a chronic illness such as HIV/AIDS, we need all the help we can get. The help of a Power greater than ourselves is available to us through prayer (talking to our Higher Power) and meditation (listening to our Higher Power). By praying and meditating in our daily lives, we keep a channel open to our Higher Power. We can rely on that Power's strength to help us at any time as we deal with the challenges of our disease.

Step Eleven calls for us to follow our Higher Power's will as it is revealed to us through prayer and meditation. Once we believe we are trying to do our Higher Power's will, we can ask for the strength to carry that out. When we do not feel like taking our medicine, exercising, or eating properly, we can ask for encouragement. When we have a compulsion to use intraveneous drugs, we can ask our Higher Power to take it away. Our Higher Power is always with us and willing to come to our aid.

It's important for us to remember that although we have turned over care of our disease to a Higher Power, we need to cooperate with that Power. By listening to others who share our condition, learning about our disease, and adhering to our doctors' advice, we are doing what is necessary to care for our HIV/AIDS and ourselves as our Higher Power wishes us to. And in so doing we will be better able to receive the strength that Power wants to provide.

The Importance of Prayer and Meditation

Medical science has demonstrated that prayer and meditation have a beneficial effect on our health (see pages xvii–xviii). These practices do this by helping us develop a closer relationship with our Higher Power, an improved "spirit consciousness."

Prayer is talking to our Higher Power. Meditation is listening to our Higher Power. Prayer and meditation don't come easily to everyone. As with most things, the more we do it, the better we get. Those who have cultivated a close relationship with their Higher Power can suggest ways that we, too, can pray and meditate. We need to seek out such people and consult them or read books on how to pray and meditate.

Perhaps the most often-heard recommendation is to have a quiet time each morning during which we ask our Higher Power for the strength to manage our HIV/AIDS that day and a similar interlude each night when we thank our Higher Power for helping us to live another day with our chronic illness.

Many people meditate at least thirty minutes a day—a time we may need to work up to. Meditation involves quieting the mind. We can begin meditating by getting in a comfortable position, closing our eyes, and focusing on a word, such as *peace.* At first, many thoughts of what we "should" be doing enter our minds, but we learn to release them. When our minds are quiet, we are able to get in touch with our inner selves and to listen to our Higher Power. Afterward, sometimes miraculously, answers to our problems will just come to us.

The strength we need to cope with our chronic illness comes from communicating with our Higher Power in prayer and meditation. We must actively seek out spirit communication with our Higher Power. This is a matter directly between us and that Power. From direct communication comes life, joy, peace, and spiritual healing.

Step Twelve: Carrying the Message

Having had a spiritual awakening as the result of these steps, we tried to carry our message to others with our condition and to practice these principles in all our affairs.

By the time we reach Step Twelve, we've changed. The compulsion to deny our disease and to engage in behaviors that not only caused it but also made it worse has been lifted—not by our own power, but by a Power greater than ourselves. This in itself is a spiritual awakening that will help us as we contend with our disease.

If we've worked the Steps, we have the gift of being able to manage our chronic illness. If we haven't worked the program, we now know we have the tools.

Truly one of the best ways to keep this gift is to give it away. We have experience, strength, and hope that we can share with others. We let ourselves be used as a channel for a Higher Power to work through. We can now partake in the joy of helping others to live healthier, happier, and longer lives.

One way we might "give it away" is to make ourselves available as volunteers to HIV/AIDS hotlines (refer to the appendix for contact information) or to those who organize HIV/AIDS prevention or safe-sex campaigns. Or we might provide comfort and company to people with HIV/AIDS living in hospices or convalescent homes. If we attend AIDS support group meetings or Narcotics Anonymous meetings, we can help make the coffee, set up beforehand, and clean up afterward.

If a member of our support group seems to be dwelling on the negative aspects of his or her life, we might spend some time with this person and try to lend a sympathetic ear and an encouraging word.

Whether or not we find an organized support group, we need to seek out and make friends with two or more people with HIV/AIDS. We need to have breakfast or lunch with them often, phone them regularly, and talk. We can praise their efforts and celebrate their successes (no matter how small) and let them do the same for us.

If we practice the principles of this Twelve Step program in all our affairs, we will likely realize our full physical potential with this disease and an abundance of spirit. We live as our Higher Power intends us to—happy, joyous, and free.

On Spiritual Awakenings

For those unfamiliar with Twelve Step programs, the term "spiritual awakening" can be the subject of confusion. Many people assume that a spiritual awakening is by definition a cataclysmic occurrence—an opening of the heavens accompanied by a chorus of hallelujahs. In the absence of such an event, some of us might assume the program isn't working for us. But instant and dramatic conversions to spirit consciousness are not what the Twelve Steps are predicated on. Although such transformations take place, they are by no means the rule. Most spiritual awakenings are simple— very simple—yet the feeling we leave with is profound. We feel enlightened and in awe.

A spiritual awakening could be as simple as a thought we have while walking through the woods or watching a child. It could be suddenly seeing ourselves or others in a totally different light. It could be running into someone who gives us the answer to the question we've been asking ourselves.

A person may have one big spiritual awakening, but most people have many smaller-scale awakenings. As the Twelve Steps become our guide to living well with HIV/AIDS and as we develop a relationship with a Power greater than ourselves who loves us and cares for us, we come to an understanding of what is truly meant by the words *spiritual awakening.*

Step by Step

We're now aware of the Twelve Steps and what they mean. They aren't always easy to accept or understand because the program, as we have heard, is *simple* but not *easy*. We pause on landings along the way: after the first three Steps (acceptance, hope, faith); after Steps Four through Seven (inner housecleaning); again after Eight and Nine (relationships with other people); and finally after the summing-up (Steps Ten, Eleven, and Twelve). We continue to make important discoveries about our inner selves, about how we relate to others, and about our spiritual links to a Higher Power.

We strive for progress, not perfection. We go back over the Steps again and again, understanding them a little better each time. We know, though, that we have the tools we need to transcend the emotional pain of our chronic illness. In the face of overwhelming odds, we move forward.

These are our own personal miracles, for which we are endlessly grateful.

CHAPTER THREE

Medical Interventions for HIV/AIDS

By practicing the principles of a Twelve Step program in your daily affairs, you will come to experience the serenity you will need to live the rest of your life with HIV and AIDS. Above all, you will have learned to turn over your disease to the care of a Higher Power. You are now working with that Power.

Serenity doesn't mean apathy. Part of your responsibility to your Higher Power is to do all that is necessary to care for yourself. Remember, AIDS isn't a death sentence. Many people with HIV are alive and well fifteen years after being diagnosed.

People with HIV and AIDS benefit by taking a proactive approach to their disease. Being proactive means

- finding the right kind of medical care
- taking steps immediately to maintain or improve your overall health

• starting treatment *before* physical symptoms occur

It's also important to take steps to cope with the emotional and psychological challenges of a chronic illness. This aspect will be covered in the next chapter.

Choosing a Doctor

HIV is a complicated disease, and so is the way it is treated. Treatments change frequently, and many different choices need to be made at every stage of the disease. Choosing a doctor who's right for you is one of the most important decisions you will have to make early on. Many factors go into this decision.

First Things First

If your primary care doctor has no expertise with HIV, the choice becomes whether to use an HIV doctor to handle your HIV problems and your primary care doctor for non-HIV-related conditions or to turn over all your medical needs to a doctor who specializes in HIV. Your decision depends on the relationship you have with your primary care physician. If you have a good relationship with that person, you may decide to continue to see him or her in addition to an HIV specialist. On the other hand, if your relationship is not particularly strong, then by all means consider turning your complete medical care over to a physician with experience in treating HIV and AIDS at all stages.

Like Minds

It's important to choose an HIV/AIDS specialist who shares your philosophy toward treatment. Some doctors are more conservative, preferring established ways of treating the disease. Others are willing to try newer and more experimental approaches. One doctor may be tremendously positive, always looking on the bright side, while the next may take a stringently realistic, or more pessimistic, view.

Some doctors believe in complementary and alternative strategies such as herbal treatments and yoga, while others frown on such approaches, advocating only Western medicine.

The more comfortable you are with your doctor's approach to treating HIV and AIDS, the easier it will be for you to get the kind of treatment you want, and the easier it will be for you to stick with it.

Is the Doctor In?

Availability is another important issue. It doesn't matter how good the doctor is if you can't schedule an appointment for months to come. Ask the doctor or the receptionist how long it generally takes to get an appointment.

The kind of insurance coverage you have may restrict your choice of a doctor. The doctor you want may not be on the list provided by your HMO or other insurance plan. Make sure you know beforehand how you are going to pay for your doctor's services.

If it's hard to get an appointment, you can use other doctors to treat your non-HIV/AIDS needs. But always use a specialist to manage your HIV and AIDS.

Private Lives

Many people prefer to keep their HIV status confidential. If that applies to you, consider choosing an HIV doctor in another town. It's up to you to find the right balance between convenience and confidentiality.

Make It a Partnership

Your doctor needs all the health information available about you to provide you with the most effective treatment. Medical records are a priority; these may have to be transferred from another doctor's office. Your new doctor will want to perform tests to get baseline information that can be used to gauge future improvements or setbacks, so cooperate fully and make yourself available. It's also important to be completely honest with your doctor, as your lifestyle may make a difference to your health care. Tell your doctor if you go back to using drugs or abusing alcohol, for instance, or if you are neglecting your drug therapy.

Making Changes

Your health needs will change over time. That is the nature of chronic disease. Furthermore, the way you look at treatment for your HIV and AIDS may evolve. While there is something to be said for continuity of treatment, you always have the right to change physicians.

Your First Appointment

The first time you see an HIV/AIDS doctor after testing positive, your doctor will take a medical history, ask a number of questions, perform a full physical, draw blood, and do a tuberculosis (TB) skin test and other tests. You will probably get some immunization shots. Tell your doctor about any health problems you are having so you can be treated for them.

Before you go for this appointment, write down a list of questions you have for your doctor about HIV and AIDS treatment, such as

- what kinds of medications you'll have to take
- how to cope with the side effects of these drugs
- where to get help quitting smoking, drugs, or alcohol

The blood your doctor draws for testing provides important information about your disease. One test tells how many CD4+ cells you have. CD4+ cells, you recall, are those cells in your body that fight viruses such as HIV. Another important blood test is *viral load testing,* which measures how much HIV is in your blood. Viral load tests help predict what will happen next with your HIV infection if you don't have treatment. Along with CD4+ cell counts, viral load tests help to determine when to start and when to change your drug therapies.

It's important that you keep your follow-up appointments. At these follow-ups, you and your doctor can discuss your test results and talk about starting drug treatments.

Working with Your Physician

Many aspects of your life change after you test positive for HIV. One thing that will probably change is your relationship with the medical profession. Like many others with HIV, you may start taking a much more assertive approach toward your medical care. This change can cause problems unless you learn to work with your doctor (and vice versa) and other practitioners. Usually you and your doctor are trying to find out what works from among a variety of available but imperfect treatments. Just as there is no single treatment therapy accepted by everyone with HIV/AIDS, there is no established position by the medical profession on how to treat the virus.

Three major factors have changed the patient-physician relationship:

- Growing numbers of people with HIV/AIDS are frustrated with the perceived lack of progress in treating the disease and are choosing more assertive treatment approaches, even if this means using unconventional treatments they prescribe themselves.
- Admitted uncertainty exists among physicians as to what their response should be to requests for non-FDA-approved medications and therapies; although not all doctors are completely opposed in principle to unconventional approaches, many physicians will condone their use.
- As part of their personal empowerment, many people with HIV/AIDS are taking an assertive role in their treatment, thus altering the traditional doctor-patient relationship.

The following paragraphs describe ways you can make your relationship with your doctor a productive one.

Do Your Homework

Find out as much as you can about HIV/AIDS before your first appointment and stay updated. Doctors rarely have time to discuss the fundamentals with their patients, so you'll be better able to understand the more advanced topics your doctor raises if you know the basics.

The limited time you have with your doctor should be spent focusing on the most important issues, so write down your questions ahead of time. Your preparation might include bringing along literature about any particular treatments you may be considering so they can be discussed.

Discuss and Settle on a Relationship Style with Your Doctor

People prefer different ways of interacting with their physicians. Some feel more secure if their doctors adopt an authoritative approach. Others prefer a partnership wherein patient and doctor make decisions together. Still others want to make all the decisions about treatment themselves, using the doctor merely as a consultant who will write prescriptions. Discuss the relationship style you want with your doctor so there is no confusion later on.

Communicate in a Spirit of Respect

Your beliefs on treatment may differ from those of your doctor. These differences may provoke disputes if you decide you want to use unconventional medications or therapies. The doctor may not reject such treatments or therapies, but he or she may not feel comfortable condoning your use of them. It's important that you learn how to talk to one another about this issue.

When unconventional treatments are discussed, certain aspects of the traditional patient-doctor relationship may be reversed. You may be more knowledgeable on these treatments than your physician. It's important to avoid confrontational attitudes when discussing the use of unconventional treatments. This requires a well-planned visit to your doctor in which adequate time for discussion is scheduled.

When the time is available and scheduled, you should discuss with your doctor what you know about a particular treatment and why you have decided to use it, making it clear from the outset that you welcome your doctor's input.

When requesting prescriptions for approved medications, a friendly but firm request is usually received best. If your doctor refuses to prescribe a medication, ask for an explanation in clear terms as to why he or she opposes use of the drug. Remember that your doctor's concerns and beliefs deserve respect, even if you don't agree with them.

Whether or not agreement is reached on the use of a particular treatment, you should secure proper monitoring of the treatment's effects. In turn, you should heed reasonable warnings suggested by the monitoring process.

Maintain All-Around Health

A healthy body is better able to fight illness. The most important components of a program to maintain overall health after being diagnosed with HIV are to eat well, exercise, reduce stress in your life, and quit using alcohol, illegal drugs, and nicotine. Numerous resources are available to help you eat better and exercise more. Later on in the progression of your disease, the issue with respect to nutrition becomes eating *enough,* and this will be addressed in chapter 5. Stress management techniques for people with HIV and AIDS will be described in chapter 4.

Abusing alcohol and drugs can impair your body's ability to fight HIV. If you think you will have a problem quitting alcohol and other drugs, seek help. Twelve Step support groups such as Alcoholics Anonymous and Narcotics Anonymous have had enormous success in helping people stay away from alcohol and other drugs one day at a time.

The Twelve Steps can also serve as key tools to quitting smoking. Nicotine Anonymous, a Twelve Step mutual-help support group, can be the starting point for smokers trying to quit or can serve as continuing care for people who complete an inpatient or outpatient smoking cessation program. If there is no listing for Nicotine Anonymous in your local telephone book, check the organization's detailed Internet site for a meeting convenient to where you live or work (www.nicotine-anonymous.org).

Substance Abuse and HIV/AIDS

If you have substance abuse issues, testing HIV-positive provides an opportunity to address your addiction. All-around health and the strength of your immune system are improved when you avoid these substances. Whatever your addiction, though, quitting can be one of the most difficult challenges you will face. Addiction is its own life-threatening illness.

Smoking cigarettes is associated with an increased incidence of Pneumocystis carinii pneumonia (PCP), as well as more frequent cases of cryptococcal meningitis (a fungal infection). Quitting smoking restores your lungs' ability to cleanse themselves within just a few weeks, and, over time, lung function continues to improve.

Smoking marijuana also harms your lungs. Marijuana is a highly addictive substance and illegal in all states except California, where the use of "medicinal" marijuana is legal. (One effect of marijuana is that it stimulates the appetite.) Regardless, using marijuana to treat chronic illnesses is highly controversial.

Chronic use or abuse of alcohol and other drugs poisons the same organs that HIV attacks (brain, liver, and immune cells). Studies show that cocaine and narcotics may encourage the AIDS virus to replicate. In many cases, when people with HIV/AIDS quit alcohol or other drugs, their health improves dramatically. This improvement is frequently reflected in their higher CD4+ counts.

Drug Treatments for HIV/AIDS

The most important drugs used to treat HIV and AIDS patients are those that fight the virus; those that boost the immune system; and those that fight opportunistic infections.

Drugs to Fight the Virus (Antivirals[1])

HIV attacks and damages the immune system. Antiviral drugs can help slow the spread of the virus. By

---

1. Antivirals are sometimes called "antiretrovirals."

themselves, none of these drugs work for an extended period; but used together in careful combinations, they can suppress HIV for many years and extend life expectancy. Antiviral drugs for HIV kill parts of the virus and thereby slow the progression of the disease. To understand how the various classes of antiviral drugs work, you have to understand the life cycle of HIV.

1. HIV attaches to a cell.
2. HIV infects the cell.
3. The HIV genetic code (RNA) is changed into DNA by the reverse transcriptase enzyme.
4. The HIV DNA is built into the infected cell's DNA by the integrase enzyme.
5. When the infected cell reproduces, it activates the HIV DNA, which makes the raw material for new AIDS viruses.
6. Packets of material for a new virus come together and push out of the infected cell.
7. The new viruses mature: the protease enzyme cuts raw materials and assembles them into a functioning virus.

Each class of antiviral drugs attacks the virus at a different stage in its life cycle.

Nucleoside reverse transcriptase inhibitors, nicknamed "nukes," were the first class of antiviral drugs.

They work by blocking step 3 in the HIV life cycle, when the genetic material is converted from RNA to DNA.

Non-nucleoside reverse transcriptase inhibitors also block step 3 but in a different way. They are nicknamed "non-nukes" and sometimes abbreviated to NNRTIs.

Protease inhibitors, the newest class of drugs to fight the virus, have generated much excitement. These drugs block step 7, where the raw material for the new AIDS virus is cut into different pieces.

Approved Antivirals

Nucleoside reverse transcriptase inhibitors—seven have been approved:

- *AZT (ZDV, zidovudine, Retrovir)*
- *didanosine (ddI, Videx)*
- *zalcitabine (ddC, Hivid)*
- *stavudine (d4T, Zerit)*
- *lamivudine (3TC, Epivir)*
- *abacavir (Ziagen)*
- *Combivir (3TC and AZT)*

Non-nucleoside reverse transcriptase inhibitors—three have been approved:

- *nevirapine (NVP, Viramune)*
- *delavirdine (DLV, Rescriptor)*
- *efavirenz (EFV, Sustiva)*

Protease inhibitors—five have been approved:

- *saquinavir (SQV, Invirase, Fortovase)*
- *indinavir (IDV, Crixivan)*
- *ritonavir (RTV, Norvir)*
- *nelfinavir (NFV, Viracept)*
- *amprenavir (APV, Agenerase)*

Taking Antiviral Drugs Properly[2]

The following information is from the New Mexico AIDS InfoNet, a project of the New Mexico AIDS Education and Training Center in the Infectious Diseases Division of the University of New Mexico School of Medicine.

This particular information concerns antiviral drugs—dosages, storage, side effects, and warnings about reactions with other drugs. Only "nukes," NNRTIs, and protease inhibitors are discussed, as these are the only three approved classes of antiviral drugs on the market.

2. Used with permission from the New Mexico AIDS InfoNet.

Nucleoside Reverse Transcriptase Inhibitors (Nukes)

Drug	Daily Pills (Adults)	How to Take & Store	Side Effects	Notes
abacavir (Ziagen)	2 (300 mg): 1, 2x/day)	No food restrictions.	Hypersensitivity reaction in 5% of patients.	
AZT (Retrovir)	6 (100 mg: 2, 3x/day) or 2 (300 mg: 1, 2x/day)	No food restrictions.	Anemia, headache, fatigue, muscle aches, bone marrow toxicity.	Don't combine with d4T.
ddI (Videx)	4 (100 mg: 2, 2x/day or 4, 1x/day)	Chew or dissolve in water; take on an empty stomach; not within 1 hour of indinavir or 2 hours of ritonavir.	Diarrhea, pancreatitis, abdominal pain, neuropathy, nausea, vomiting.	Don't combine with ddC.
ddC (Hivid)	3 (0.75 mg: 1, 3x/day)	Take on an empty stomach. Don't take with antacids.	Peripheral neuropathy, rash, mouth ulcers, sore throat, coughing.	Don't combine with ddI.
d4T (Zerit)	2 (40 mg: 1, 2x/day)	No food restrictions.	Peripheral neuropathy, headache, chills and fever, diarrhea, nausea.	Don't combine with AZT.
3TC (Epivir)	2 (150 mg: 1, 2x/day)	No food restrictions.	Nausea, vomiting, fatigue, headaches.	Can reverse resistance to AZT.
Combivir	2 (150 mg 3TC + 300 mg AZT: 1, 2x/day)	No food restrictions.	See AZT and 3TC above.	Combines AZT and 3TC in a single twice-daily pill.

	Drug	Daily Pills (Adults)	How to Take & Store	Side Effects	Notes
Non-Nucleoside Reverse Transcriptase Inhibitors (NNRTIs or Non-Nukes)	delavirdine (Rescriptor)	12 (100 mg: 4, 3x/day)	No food restrictions. Can be dissolved in water. Take 1 hour apart from ddI or antacids.	Skin rash, nausea, diarrhea, vomiting, headache, fatigue.	Serious interactions with many other drugs.*
	efavirenz (Sustiva)	3 (200 mg: 3, 1x/day)	No food restrictions, but avoid a high-fat meal. Take before going to sleep.	Rash, nausea, dizziness, diarrhea, headache, insomnia.	
	nevirapine (Viramune)	2 (200 mg: 1, 2x/day)	No food restrictions.	Skin rash, fever, headache, nausea.	

*Protease inhibitors and NNRTIs are metabolized by the liver, as are many other commonly used drugs. Drug interactions can cause large increases or decreases in the blood levels of drugs you are taking, leading to underdoses that are ineffective, or overdoses that can be fatal. Make sure your physician knows about all medications you are taking.

	Drug	Daily Pills (Adults)	How to Take & Store	Side Effects	Notes
Protease Inhibitors	amprenavir (Agenerase)	16 (150 mg: 8, 2x/day)	Take with or without food. Avoid high-fat meals. Don't take within 1 hour of antacids.	Nausea, diarrhea, vomiting, rash, numbness around mouth, abdominal pain.	Serious interactions with many other drugs.*
	indinavir (Crixivan)	8 (400 mg: 2, every 8 hours, not just 3x/day)	Take with lots of water, on empty stomach, or with low-fat snack. Keep cool and dry.	Headache, nausea, abdominal pain, kidney stones.	
	nelfinavir (Viracept)	9 (250 mg: 3, 3x/day)	Take with meals or a snack.	Diarrhea, nausea, gas, abdominal pain, weakness.	
	ritonavir (Norvir)	12 (100 mg: 6, 2x/day)	Take with a full meal. Keep refrigerated. Take 2 hours apart from ddI.	Nausea, vomiting, diarrhea, tingling and numbness around mouth.	
	saquinavir soft gel (Fortovase)	18 (200 mg: 6, 3x/day)	Take with high-fat food. Refrigerate in hot climates.	Minimal nausea, diarrhea, abdominal discomfort.	

*Protease inhibitors and NNRTIs are metabolized by the liver, as are many other commonly used drugs. Drug interactions can cause large increases or decreases in the blood levels of drugs you are taking, leading to underdoses that are ineffective, or overdoses that can be fatal. Make sure your physician knows about all medications you are taking.

How Are Antivirals Used to Fight HIV?

If only one antiviral drug is taken, a mutation that can survive the drug eventually develops. If two drugs are used, a mutant has to overcome both drugs simultaneously. And if three drugs are prescribed—especially if they attack the HIV at different points in its life cycle—it is hard for a mutation to develop that can sidestep all three drugs at one time. Studies show that resistance takes much longer to develop when using a triple-drug combination. Using just one antiviral drug is considered outdated.

Do Antivirals Cure HIV/AIDS?

As mentioned, a viral load test measures the amount of HIV in your blood. The lower the viral load, the longer you will stay healthy. Triple-drug combinations have lowered some people's viral loads to a level that is undetectable. This doesn't mean, however, that the virus has been driven from their bodies. The virus is "hiding" and multiplying very slowly.

At one time doctors thought that effective drug therapy could eventually kill all of the virus in your body. This now seems improbable. It may be possible to reduce the amount of the virus in your body and to repair your immune system so significantly that you could stop taking antiviral drugs.

When to Start Treatment

When to start antiviral medication has been the subject of strenuous debate. Some researchers believe it's essential to start taking antivirals as soon as the virus is diagnosed, regardless of whether tests reveal your CD4+ count is falling, whether your viral load is high or rising, and whether you have symptoms. The argument is that waiting encourages the virus to spread and infect other areas of your body. This school of thought, taken to its extreme, holds that bombarding HIV with a variety of antiviral medications soon after initial infection occurs eradicates the virus; but, so far, this has not worked. If this approach someday proves effective, then the question of when to start treatment will have been answered.

Another argument in favor of early antiviral drug treatment is that it prevents the loss of important parts of the immune system. Because researchers don't know exactly when the loss of such cells takes place, it is still difficult to know the right time to start.

Some researchers argue that it is better to start drug treatment later because none of the medications presently available work indefinitely. They contend that it is necessary to save the drugs for a time when the virus can cause more damage. They believe that prescribing drugs very early on will "use up" their effectiveness before they are really needed.

Even those researchers who argue that drug interventions should begin later on in the course of the disease recommend starting to take medications before significant damage to the immune system occurs.

Right now there are no set guidelines on when to start treatment. Answers will be available when clinical studies have been completed. So for now it comes down to personal choice. Discuss your options with your doctor.

Keep in mind that researchers are unanimous in advocating that antiviral drugs begin in the following cases:

- when symptoms exist
- when CD4+ count is falling
- when viral load is high

Using Antivirals: The Basics

Guidelines for using antiviral drugs keep changing. There are legitimate reasons why. In the past few years, many new antivirals have been developed. Ongoing research constantly changes doctors' understanding of the most effective way to use these drugs to fight HIV.

What follows are the most up-to-date guidelines.

When Should Viral Load Testing Be Done?

Viral load testing provides vital information for decisions on antiviral therapy. Testing viral load is recommended in the following situations:

- before starting or changing medications, to get a reference value
- about two to eight weeks after starting or changing medications, to see if the new drugs are working
- every three or four months, to make sure the medications are still working; or, for patients who aren't taking medications, to help decide when to start

What Drugs Should Be Used at First?

At the start of antiviral drug therapy, current guidelines recommend using two nucleoside reverse transcriptase inhibitors (nukes) plus one of the following:

- a single protease inhibitor
- a combination of ritonavir and saquinavir
- the NNRTI efavirenz (Sustiva)

A less effective combination would be two nukes plus nevirapine or delavirdine or the triple-nuke combination of AZT, 3TC, and abacavir. Current guidelines discourage the use of a single drug (monotherapy) or just two nukes.

When Should Treatment Be Interrupted?

It may be necessary to interrupt treatment for several reasons:

- if you can't tolerate the side effects
- if there's a bad interaction between drugs
- if you get pregnant (antivirals shouldn't be taken during the first three months of pregnancy)

If you have to interrupt your antiviral therapy, you should stop using all the drugs at the same time, and restart them *all* at the same time. This will reduce the risk of the HIV developing resistance to the medications.

When Should Treatment Change?

The goal of antiviral therapy is to reduce viral load to undetectable levels and keep it there. Treatment should be changed if it doesn't appear to be working or if you can't tolerate the drugs you're using.

Treatment is usually considered to have failed if within four weeks viral load hasn't dropped by 70 to 80 percent. Within six months, the viral load should be undetectable. If these goals haven't been reached, change your treatment.

Other signs of treatment failure include one or more of the following:

- an increase in viral load from undetectable to detectable levels or to more than three times its lowest level on the drugs being used
- a continuing drop in CD4+ cells
- a new AIDS-related illness

What Should Change Involve?

Deciding what to change should be based on several factors: the reason for changing; how sick you are; medications you've used previously; other drugs available; side effects you've had; and other medications being used.

If you're changing your drug treatment because of drug intolerance, your doctor may reduce the dose of the drug causing the problems or replace it with one or more drugs from the same class and of the same strength.

If you're changing due to failure of the particular therapy, your doctor may consider prescribing the following:

- Use at least two new drugs, preferably an entirely new combination.
- Avoid using any drug you have used before.
- Do not switch to any drug that has shown cross-resistance with a drug now being used; for instance, don't switch between ritonavir and indinavir or between nevirapine and delavirdine.

If options for change are few and viral load was reduced, your doctor may recommend that you not change medication. Another choice may be to combine two protease inhibitors or a protease inhibitor and an NNRTI.

The Future of Antiviral Drugs

New drugs to fight HIV are being developed in all three classes. Medical scientists are also trying to develop new types of drugs that will interfere with the AIDS virus at different points in its life cycle.

These are some of the more promising antiviral drugs in development:

- *Integrase inhibitors:* This class of drugs blocks the action of integrase, an enzyme that inserts the viral DNA into the infected cell's DNA strands. No integrase inhibitors have been approved yet. One drug, AR-177 (Zintevir), is in phase I human trials.
- *Fusion inhibitors:* This class of drugs prevents HIV from attaching to a cell. No fusion inhibitors have been approved yet. Four fusion inhibitors are in human trials: AMD-3100, in phase II trials; T-20 (Pentafuside), in phase II trials; FP21399, in phase I trials; and PRO 452, in phase I/II trials.
- *Antisense drugs:* This class of drugs is a mirror image of part of the HIV genetic code that locks onto the virus to prevent it from functioning. One antisense drug, HGTV43, is in phase I trials.

Drugs to Boost the Immune System

The purpose of *immune modulating medications* is to increase the number of cells that help fight viruses (especially CD4+ cells), restore balance to the immune system, and/or reduce the harm done by cells damaged by the virus.

Not enough is known about the immune system, however, to make these kinds of therapies particularly effective. Boosting the immune system isn't as easy as some people make it sound—especially when it comes to fighting a powerful and ingenious virus such as HIV. It is difficult to strengthen a particular part of the immune system without weakening another. The bottom line is that no matter what immune modulating medications are used, the body's defense system nearly always succumbs to the virus. Straightforward as it may sound, boosting the immune system is the least promising of the treatments presently available.

Interleukin 2 (Il-2, Aldesleukin, Proleukin) is in phase II/III trials; Reticulose is in phase III trials; and Multikine is in phase I trials. Also, an inactivated virus preparation, HIV-1 Immunogen (Remune), is in phase III trials.

Drugs to Fight Opportunistic Infections

Once tests show that your immune system has been damaged to a particular degree, it becomes necessary to try to prevent the occurrence or recurrence of the most common opportunistic infections. Preventive drug treatment is becoming available for many opportunistic infections.

Taking a drug to prevent a certain opportunistic infection should be considered when CD4+ counts approach a danger zone for that infection. For instance, the risk of Pneumocystis carinii pneumonia (PCP) gets much higher when the CD4+ count drops below 300, while the risk for cytomegalovirus (CMV) is greater when it drops below 100. Careful and timely use of medication can prevent PCP altogether. Because tuberculosis (TB) is prevalent in people with HIV, regular testing and immunizations are recommended.

When your HIV becomes advanced, it is usually necessary to try to treat or prevent several opportunistic infections at the same time. Choosing which medications to take can be a challenge because certain drugs interact with each other. You will need to be informed and work carefully with your doctor to sort this out.

Finding Better HIV/AIDS Treatments: You Can Help[3]

Doctors have learned a great deal in a short time about how to help people with HIV. But more and better drugs are needed. Research studies known as "clinical trials" are a key step to finding them.

What Are Clinical Trials?

A new drug goes through careful testing before doctors use it to treat people who are sick. First, it is tested in labs and in animals. If these tests show promise, researchers test the drug in people. When a drug is tested in people, the test is called a clinical trial. These tests show whether a new drug is safe in people and whether it helps them to get better.

Clinical trials have already helped people with AIDS. Not long ago, we had almost no drugs to treat people who have HIV. Today, we have drugs that

- *help people who have AIDS, or who have some signs of AIDS, live longer*
- *help people who have HIV, but who are not yet sick, stay well longer*

3. From information provided by the Office of Communications and Public Liaison, National Institute of Allergy and Infectious Diseases, National Institutes of Health, Bethesda, MD 20892.

- *treat or prevent problems caused by infections related to AIDS, such as pneumonia and blindness*

These drugs were proved to work because people with HIV helped test them.

How Can You Help?

Most studies today compare a new drug or set of drugs with the one now being used to see which treatment works better.

Researchers are looking for men, women, and children to help test new drugs for HIV. You may want to think about joining a study if you

- *have HIV*
- *have some early symptoms of AIDS, such as fever, swollen glands, or diarrhea*
- *have AIDS*

As one AIDS patient named Maria said, "Being in a study means making some sacrifices, keeping up your end of the bargain. It's worth it to me. But you should get all the facts before you decide."

Clinical Trials: Pros and Cons

Pros:

- *People in a study may be the first to be helped, if a new drug is shown to work.*

- *People in a study get very good health care.*
- *Some of your medical costs are covered.*
- *Joining means taking action to try to help yourself.*
- *You have a chance to help others with HIV.*

Cons:

- *A study may involve a great deal of time, tests, and changes in your schedule.*
- *The new treatment may not work, or it may not help you as much as it helps others.*
- *The treatment may be harmful; it could make you worse instead of better.*
- *The drug may have side effects that make you feel worse.*

Many studies are done in clinics at large hospitals. Most people who take part live nearby. Others move or travel to the clinics to receive their treatment. In some cases, people can also join research studies at smaller clinics near where they live.

All studies have rules about who can take part. Before you can join, you will first have some medical tests to be sure you are right for the study.

How to Find Out More

Where should you go to find out more about studies that you might join or to get more information about HIV?

- *Your doctor or clinic. This is the place to start to learn about studies in your area.*
- *AIDS Clinical Trials Information Service (ACTIS). This is a call-in service where trained staff will tell you about studies for people who have HIV. Your call and your name will be kept private. You can ask for a list of new drugs being tested, where the trials are, and who is doing the studies. English and Spanish are spoken. Call toll-free (800) TRIALS-A (800-874-2572). Lines are open Monday through Friday, 9:00 A.M. to 7:00 P.M. eastern time.*
- *HIV/AIDS Trials Information Service. You can find out about government-approved treatments for HIV by calling (800) HIV-0440 (800-448-0440). For hearing-impaired access, call (800) 243-7012. The service is open Monday through Friday, 9:00 A.M. to 7:00 P.M. eastern time.*
- *The National AIDS Hotline. The hotline can give you basic facts about AIDS as well as tell you about AIDS support groups, clinics,*

and other help in your area. Call toll-free (800) 342-AIDS (800-342-2437). Spanish-speaking callers can dial (800) 344-SIDA (800-344-7432). For hearing-impaired access, call (800) AIDS-TTY (800-243-7889). Lines are open seven days a week, twenty-four hours a day.

CHAPTER FOUR

Daily Living with HIV/AIDS

Among the most common emotional and psychological symptoms of having a chronic condition such as HIV and AIDS are depression, anger, and fear and anxiety. It's important to know how to recognize and cope with these symptoms.

Recognizing Depression

Learning you have HIV hits hard. The knowledge that your life will never again be the same can cause feelings of great loss. It's common for people diagnosed with HIV to experience feelings of emptiness, hopelessness, and sadness. Then there is the loss of self-esteem—this may surface as feelings of uselessness and perhaps even guilt and shame about having HIV/AIDS. All these emotions are consistent with depression. Signs that you have depression include a persistent feeling of sadness, not sleeping properly, loss of interest in activities you once enjoyed, and the inability to concentrate.

Depression may be short-term or could become severe—a condition known as *major depressive disorder.* If symptoms persist for longer than two weeks or become noticeably more severe, tell your doctor. He or she may refer you to a mental health professional or prescribe antidepressant medication. Definitely speak to your doctor if you answer yes to four or more of the following questions:

- Do you feel sad, anxious, hopeless, or on the verge of tears for much of the day, every day?
- Have you lost interest in enjoyable activities such as eating, sex, and socializing?
- Are you eating more or less than usual? Have you gained or lost a significant amount of weight?
- Do you feel agitated, fidget constantly, or find yourself incapable of staying still?
- Are you always weary? Are you too fatigued to take on even small chores?
- Are you having problems concentrating?
- Have you had thoughts of wanting to die?

Sometimes people with HIV/AIDS have depression caused by one of the medications they are taking. Because the depression is probably not going to be permanent, antidepressants are usually not prescribed in such cases. However, certain people experience depression caused by chemical changes in their bodies that may require antidepressants to alleviate. The doctor treating your HIV/AIDS needs to know about any antidepressants you are taking.

Recognizing Anger

It doesn't matter how you became infected with HIV. Chances are that when you found out you have the disease, you became angry. If you got it through sexual contact, you could be angry at the person who gave it to you or angry at yourself for being promiscuous; if you got it through intravenous drug use, you may be angry at yourself or other drug addicts around you at the time; if you got it through a transfusion, you may be angry at the hospital where you had the procedure.

Recognizing Fear and Anxiety

Fear is an inevitable part of having a chronic illness, and HIV is no exception. There is the fear of not knowing how your disease will progress and how well drug treatment will work; the fear of rejection by friends and family; and the fear that HIV/AIDS could affect your employment situation. Anxiety resembles fear. It includes feelings of nervousness or tension in response to a particular situation—in this case, having the chronic illness HIV/AIDS.

These are the symptoms associated with anxiety:

Mental: Impatience, restlessness, tension, problems concentrating, difficulty sleeping, and loss of enjoyment of pleasurable activities

Physical: Dry mouth, nausea, sweating, dizziness, diarrhea, constipation, muscle aches, sexual difficulties, rapid heartbeat, and shortness of breath

Coping with Emotional and Psychological Symptoms

There are several ways to overcome the negative feelings that follow discovering you have HIV and those feelings that may arise in the course of trying to cope with your disease.

Finding Help

Participating in a Twelve Step program is one way. A Twelve Step program to cope with HIV/AIDS is described in chapter 2. "Working the Steps" has helped millions of people trying to overcome feelings of depression, anger, and fear and anxiety associated with chronic illness.

It may also be necessary to seek help from a mental health professional, especially if negative emotions start to overwhelm you. Although a stigma goes along with seeking professional help for mental health, the results can be profoundly beneficial for someone with HIV/AIDS. A therapist who counsels those with chronic illness—preferably people with HIV/AIDS—can help you find ways to cope with the emotional and psychological challenges of your disease. A therapist will help you talk regarding your concerns about your disease, show you how to get involved in enjoyable activities, and suggest ways to positively channel your energies.

A therapist can also direct you to an HIV/AIDS support group. Finding a support group is important for anyone who has HIV/AIDS. Even when you know intellectually that you are one of millions of people with HIV/AIDS, sometimes there's a tendency to think you're going through this alone.

As soon as you begin your drug regimen—or even if your doctor decides your condition is not yet severe enough that you need such therapy—you should seek out an HIV/AIDS support group. Do this even if you don't believe support groups are for you. The relief that comes from sharing thoughts, feelings, and coping strategies with people in the same position as yourself can be monumental. Don't discount the importance of these groups before you've given them a fair chance. Attend at least six meetings with an open mind before you decide whether they're for you.

A support group should meet at least once or twice

a week for one or two hours at a time. Although some people recommend that a therapist be present to guide the discussion, many groups (including Twelve Step programs such as Narcotics Anonymous) offer excellent support for their members without paid professionals present.

The role of a therapist in an HIV/AIDS support group is, in part, to make sure that the discussion does not focus on the negative. In a group without a therapist present, participants must remember that while a support group is a place to share hardships, the emphasis is on the positive progress the participants have made since starting therapy. Certain meetings should be set aside for spouses and family members to also attend.

There may be no support groups in your area, in which case think about starting one yourself. Get advice about starting a support group from a group therapist at your local community services organization.

You may decide to use the Twelve Steps as the basis for the support group you form. Why not? After all, the Steps have been used with extraordinary success by people dealing with a variety of other chronic illnesses. If you decide to make yours a Twelve Step group, learn how to run it by talking to the Alcoholics Anonymous World Services office in New York at (212) 870-3400 or by talking with someone who is very familiar with Twelve Step groups. A longtime member of Alcoholics Anonymous, Nicotine Anonymous, Overeaters Anonymous, or Al-Anon (a Twelve Step program for family members and adult children of alcoholics) would be ideal. That person might recommend you also incorporate the Twelve Traditions of AA as guidelines for how to organize your group.

If it isn't practical for you to attend or start a support group—perhaps because of your geographical location or because your AIDS is too advanced—and even if you are a regular participant in such a group, consider getting involved in an Internet "chat room" for people with HIV. Many of these are certainly available.

By communicating and interacting with others who share your disease, you may discover that having HIV/AIDS has presented you with the opportunity to address issues that would otherwise have remained unmanaged and which, having been dealt with, will make you a more complete person.

Getting Informed

A fear of the unknown is behind many of the negative feelings associated with chronic illness. So it's also important to learn as much as you can about your disease. Reading this book is a good start. There are other excellent published sources of information about HIV/AIDS, but be sure to seek out those that address the emotional and psychological issues of having a long-term disease.

If you haven't done so already, find a physician who is knowledgeable about HIV/AIDS and discuss treatment options.

Another useful source of information is the Internet. If you have a telephone line and a computer, then the vast resources of the Internet are available to you. If you don't have a computer, your local public library probably has Internet access for library patrons. Once you are online, most medical research resources on the Internet are free. Some sites take the latest medical research and "translate" it into information the ordinary person can understand. Lessons on how to use the Internet are widely available; classes may be held at your local library, senior center, or adult learning center. Keep in mind that many sites on the Internet contain dubious information, so be a discriminating "net surfer."

Learning Stress Management Techniques

Having HIV/AIDS can be very stressful. Studies show that people with HIV/AIDS benefit from some form of structured daily relaxation. Numerous studies reported at recent international AIDS conferences have shown that regular relaxation decreases depression, improves attitude, and strengthens the immune system. Conversely, high levels of stress can weaken the immune system, which can lead to increases in HIV/AIDS-related symptoms and infections.

Following are some simple ways to deal with stress:

- Exercise.
- Take time to relax with a good book, a movie, or music.
- Develop new interests, or rekindle interests in past activities (take a course).
- Interact—spend time with family and friends.
- Address a person or situation that's causing you to react stressfully.
- Join a support group.
- Learn about your disease, but don't obsess about it.

The National Institutes of Health recognizes the following methods as ways to reduce stress levels:

- prayer
- psychotherapy
- support groups
- art, music, and dance therapy
- hypnosis
- biofeedback

- yoga
- imagery

One of the most effective ways to deal with stress is prayer. Praying decreases blood pressure, heart rate, and breathing rates. The beneficial change that occurs in the human body in response to prayer is known as the "relaxation response." A short invocation known as the Serenity Prayer can be said anytime you feel stress.

> God grant me the serenity
> To accept the things I cannot change,
> The courage to change the things I can,
> And the wisdom to know the difference.

Prayer is not the only way to evoke the relaxation response. There are dozens of other relaxation techniques. Some of them, such as meditation, are centuries-old. Others, such as biofeedback, have been developed only in the last few decades. If living with HIV/AIDS is causing you extreme stress, then the more methods of relaxation you know, the better. Compare this with fitness. The more forms of exercise you can do, the easier it is to stay in shape. That's because you have different exercise modes for different situations and moods. The same goes for relaxation.

Two of the most common relaxation techniques are deep breathing and meditation.

Deep Breathing

Deep breathing is a simple and effective way to relax. It is also one of the most practical methods because you can do it almost anywhere. Deep breathing is a component of many other relaxation and meditation techniques, making it a good skill to master. Here is one breathing technique you can use:

- Sit up straight or lie flat on your back.
- Breathe in slowly through your nose and imagine you are pushing that air deep into your belly.
- Note how your belly expands as your lungs fill with air.
- Now breathe out slowly through your mouth.
- Continue breathing in this way, watching how your belly rises and falls.
- Do this twice a day for five minutes at a time.

Meditation

Like deep breathing, meditation can be done almost anywhere, although most people prefer—and beginners may need—peace, quiet, and solitude. Meditation is an intense and inward-focused concentration that allows you to focus on your senses, step back from your thoughts and feelings, and perceive each moment as a unique event. Meditation puts you in a rest state. You actually rest more deeply when meditating than when sleeping.

Generally, meditation can be classified as two different types: concentrative and mindfulness meditation.

Concentrative meditation uses a picture, word, or phrase (mantra), object (such as a candle flame), or a sensation (such as breathing) to focus the mind. If your mind begins to wander, you refocus your attention on the item you have chosen.

Mindfulness meditation is more complicated. Instead of focusing on a single sensation or object, you allow thoughts, feelings, and images to float through your mind. You let these thoughts go in and out of your mind without expressing positive or negative feelings about them.

Other forms of relaxation range from the high-tech (biofeedback, isolation tanks) to the physical (aerobic exercise, stretching). Some people find that combining several relaxation techniques—biofeedback, visualization, and psychotherapy, for instance—helps them best. Determine which relaxation techniques work best for you and make them part of your day!

Telling Others You Have HIV/AIDS

So many misconceptions exist about HIV/AIDS and there is still a stigma attached to having the disease. As a result, revealing that you have HIV/AIDS—even to close friends and family—can be a daunting prospect. Many people find they are ashamed to admit they have this disease.

It is important, however, that you tell those close to you. Their support and understanding will help you deal with the physical, emotional, and mental challenges of your chronic illness. Also, you will need their help when you are not up to performing certain tasks, such as housework or running errands, and when you need help getting to the doctor's office, eating balanced meals, and having the right medications on hand. And, of course, you need to tell others so they won't inadvertently catch the virus from you.

Whom should you tell that you have HIV/AIDS? Three recommendations are

- people you trust
- people who care about you
- people who are in a position to help you

People tend to be afraid of what they don't understand, so when you tell others you have HIV/AIDS, it is important you also provide them with solid, accurate information. Letting them read this book may be a help. In the meantime, it's important that you cover three important topics with your confidants:

- what the symptoms may be and how you might be affected
- what, if any, treatment you will be having and what the side effects of the treatment may be
- what the risk is of infecting others with HIV/AIDS[1]

HIV/AIDS in the Workplace

If telling a friend or family member that you have HIV/AIDS is difficult, then informing people at work may seem out of the question. Yet this deserves careful consideration, as you probably can and need to keep your job as you manage your disease.

In general, use the same criteria for telling your colleagues as your family: tell those whom you trust, those who care about you, and those who can help you.

What about your employer? This is a difficult question. Before you make your decision, consider how having HIV/AIDS might affect your job and ask your doctor whether you are putting others at risk in

1. Remember to stress that the risk of transmission is very low because the virus can only be transmitted through blood and that it cannot be transmitted through casual contact such as hugging, holding hands, or kissing.

your place of work. If you have HIV/AIDS, the risks of transmitting the disease to others in the workplace is usually small.

There are pros and cons to telling your boss. On the plus side, he or she will understand your situation better and may be able to help you cope and continue in your employment. But there may be a downside if your employer adopts a negative attitude. Fortunately, federal and state laws protect you. The federal Americans with Disabilities Act (ADA) protects you from being fired or pressured to quit because of your condition—so long as you can continue doing your job despite your illness. This doesn't mean you won't be fired or discriminated against if you tell people at work about your condition; it simply means you have a right to sue if your employer does not obey this law.

The ADA: A Primer[2]

Your employer cannot legally discriminate against you because you have HIV/AIDS. According to the Americans with Disabilities Act, employers cannot legally

- *limit your opportunities or status*
- *institute company policies that discriminate against you because you have HIV/AIDS*

---

2. Employers with fewer than fifteen employees are not bound by the ADA.

- *refuse to make reasonable changes to help you continue to do your job*
- *use your disease as an excuse to prevent you from doing some aspect of your job*

In addition, a prospective employer cannot ask you questions about your condition during the job interview.

To claim your rights under the ADA, you must be able to perform the essential functions of your job, and you must have told your employer about your condition.

If you believe your employer is violating the law, you can contact the local office of the Equal Employment Opportunity Commission (EEOC), which handles ADA complaints. You can also contact the Department of Justice, which operates the ADA Mediation Program, to try to resolve such problems. If you can't reach a resolution, you can still sue under the provisions of the ADA.

If you decide to reveal your condition to your employer, you need to decide whom to inform. You may want to start with the human resources or medical department, if your company has one. If you decide to tell your boss, choose a calm time at work to ask for a private moment. Try to anticipate any questions he or she might have and consider bringing along this book or an informational brochure. In particular, be ready to answer questions from your boss about how the disease might affect your job performance and what the likelihood is of transmitting the disease to your co-workers.

For specific advice on your situation, consult a lawyer in your area. A local legal/law association may be able to help you find one who specializes in disability law.

Using the Family Leave Act

The Family Medical Leave Act (FMLA) provides that if you have worked full-time for a company for a year or more, you can take up to twelve weeks of unpaid leave every year to attend to serious medical problems. The time can be taken all at once or in increments. Your spouse or another family member can also take this time if your condition is serious enough that he or she needs to care for you. Make sure you speak with your boss about the FMLA before you take any time off. In addition to the federal FMLA, many states have laws that provide similar protection.

CHAPTER FIVE

The Importance of Good Nutrition and Exercise

Developing a solid foundation for better health involves making some well-established, common-sense lifestyle choices. Among these are improving nutrition and exercising your body.

Nutrition

Nutrition is the process by which you assimilate food and use it for growth and replacing tissues. Good nutrition can be difficult to maintain when you have HIV/AIDS. On the one hand, when your body fights an infection, it uses more energy than usual, so you need to eat more than usual. On the other hand, because you don't feel well, you eat less. This discrepancy can lead to significant weight loss, even early on in the disease's progression, often before symptoms are present and when CD4+ counts are high. Furthermore, malnourishment helps the virus spread more quickly.

Good nutrition, then, is vital for anyone who has HIV/AIDS and should really be thought of along with doctor-prescribed medications as co-therapy for the disease. Good nutrition can help people with HIV and AIDS in these ways:

- prevent or delay loss of muscle mass ("wasting")
- decrease the risk and severity of opportunistic infections
- lessen the symptoms of HIV/AIDS

Eating well every day takes real commitment—but it's worth the effort. Start by discussing your diet with your doctor or nutritionist. There are plenty of excellent books and nutritional guides for people who are HIV-positive, as well as numerous online resources. Nutritional counseling is also available from a number of organizations, including local social service agencies and HIV/AIDS support services. Be sure to choose a counselor who is qualified and familiar with the specific challenges facing people with HIV. Your nutritionist will need to work in conjunction with the doctor handling your HIV. Finally, keep in mind that most of the information out there about nutrition and diet is for people trying to lose weight—at best, it isn't relevant to you if you have HIV/AIDS; at worst, it can be dangerous.

The Essentials of Eating Well

Everyone should eat a healthy diet. Healthy eating means a balanced diet containing a variety of foods that, when eaten together, provide you with all the important nutrients your body needs every day to work properly.

The Food Guide Pyramid provided by the U.S. Department of Agriculture (USDA) is an excellent guide to eating a balanced diet. It is a simplified, systematic way to ensure an adequate intake of calories and all essential nutrients. It goes beyond the "basic food groups" once promoted by nutritionists and other health professionals. The Food Guide Pyramid is based on the USDA's research on what foods Americans eat, what nutrients are in those foods, and how individuals can make the right food choices. The pyramid helps people choose what and how much to eat from each food group to keep fat and saturated-fat intake low. A diet low in fat reduces the chances of getting certain diseases and helps maintain a healthy weight. The pyramid also helps individuals learn how to spot and control the amount of sugar and salt in their diet.

Here are the basics of using the Food Guide Pyramid.

What to Eat: The Food Guide Pyramid in Brief

Bread, Cereal, Rice, and Pasta: Choose six to eleven servings of bread, cereal, rice, and other grains daily. Include some whole grains, such as whole wheat or enriched bread or bran cereal. Any one of the following is equivalent to one serving of grain:

- 1 slice of bread
- 1 ounce of ready-to-eat cereal
- ½ cup of cooked cereal, rice, or pasta

Fruit: Choose two to four servings of fruit daily, including one good source of vitamin C, such as orange juice. Any one of the following is equivalent to one serving of fruit:

- a medium banana, apple, or orange
- ½ cup of cooked, canned, or cut-up fruit
- ¾ cup of juice

Vegetable: Choose three to five servings of vegetables daily, including at least one serving of a dark leafy green or dark orange vegetable, such as

- ½ cup of cooked carrots or chopped vegetables
- 1 cup of raw, leafy vegetables such as lettuce or spinach
- ¾ cup of vegetable juice

Meat, Poultry, Fish, Dry Beans, Eggs, and Nuts:
Choose two to three servings equaling five to seven ounces daily of meat, poultry, fish, and other protein foods, such as beans, eggs, tofu, and unsalted nuts. Any one of the following is equivalent to a one-ounce portion of meat, fish, or chicken:

- 1 egg
- ½ cup of tofu
- ½ cup of cooked beans
- 2 tablespoons of peanut butter

Milk, Yogurt, and Cheese: Choose two to three servings of milk, cheese, or yogurt daily. Any one of the following is equivalent to one serving of a dairy product:

- 1 cup of milk
- 1 cup of yogurt
- 1 ½ ounces of cheese

Coping with Common Eating Problems

People with HIV/AIDS often experience problems with eating. These may be the result of the virus, opportunistic infections, or the side effects of medications. The most common problems are nausea/vomiting, diarrhea, difficulty chewing or swallowing, and loss of appetite. Following are ways to overcome these problems.

Nausea/Vomiting

Most people can't "stomach" the thought of eating when they are nauseated. But not eating well makes you sicker and will interfere with the way your body absorbs your medications, so it's important to learn ways to overcome your nausea.

The following suggestions may help you eat even when you feel nauseated:

- DO cut a lemon in half, rub it between your hands, and inhale the lemon's aroma—it'll calm your stomach and relieve nausea.
- DO eat while watching TV—it can make you forget about your nausea.
- DO eat foods that may be easier on your stomach: clear soups or broth; rice, noodles, oatmeal, or cream of wheat without butter or sauce; mashed potatoes; plain eggs, cottage cheese, or yogurt; pudding or gelatin; plain crackers, pretzels, or unbuttered popcorn; and canned fruit, fruit ices, or a chilled supplement. Try your personal comfort foods.
- DO eat and drink slowly. Breathe deeply. Relax. Take your time.

- DO eat small meals throughout the day. Try six or eight small meals instead of three big ones.
- DO drink fluids that are high in nutrients, such as juices and electrolyte replacement drinks, between meals.
- DO make sure your cooking area is well ventilated so that cooking odors don't nauseate you. If you do get nauseous, you may not want to eat right after you cook. Wait thirty minutes or so until your stomach calms down.
- DO eat cool foods instead of hot foods, which are more likely to make you feel nauseated.
- DO wear loose-fitting clothing while eating and rest afterward. But stay seated—don't lie down.
- DON'T drink before or during meals, as liquids will fill you up too fast.
- DON'T eat greasy or fried foods.
- DON'T eat foods with strong odors.
- DON'T eat sweet or spicy foods. Instead try foods that are either salty or bland. Plain crackers, pretzels, toast, or dry cereal may help relieve your nausea.
- DON'T eat hot meals when you could eat cool foods, which are less likely to make you nauseous. A sandwich may be better than a hot meal.

Remember to tell your doctor about your nausea. There are medications that can help relieve your symptoms. If one of your medicines is making you feel sick, it may be possible to reschedule your meals around specific medications.

Diarrhea

A common and serious problem among people with HIV/AIDS is diarrhea. This condition is so serious because it can cause weight loss and dehydration. Anyone who has diarrhea for longer than two days or experiences diarrhea that is unusually severe should see a doctor immediately.

Causes of diarrhea in people with HIV/AIDS range from medications, infections, food poisoning, food intolerance, and stress. Try to determine the cause of your diarrhea. There may be several minor reasons and not one major reason. Look into whether you may be lactose intolerant or whether grains such as bread or pasta are causing your problems. Ask your doctor to test you for parasites, bacteria, mycobacteria, or fungi. Whatever the cause, it is essential that you maintain an appropriate intake of food and fluids to prevent weight loss and dehydration.

Foods to eat if you have diarrhea include plain rice or noodles; oatmeal, cream of wheat, or farina with no milk or butter; potatoes without butter or gravy; or plain bread, toast, or crackers. If you wish, add sugar, jelly, or syrup to these foods. You might also try skinless chicken or turkey; low-fat meats and fish; hard-boiled eggs; smooth peanut butter; low-fat cheese or yogurt; applesauce, bananas, and pureed vegetables; and canned fruits and grape, orange, cranberry, peach, and apricot juices and nectars. Instead of high-fiber fruits, eat bananas, applesauce, or canned or cooked fruits—even baby food.

Eat foods at or near room temperature. Eat frequent small meals—six or eight small meals will be easier to digest than three big ones.

Foods to avoid if you have diarrhea include high-fiber foods such as raw fruits and vegetables (especially those with skins and seeds), nuts, whole grains, and corn. Also stay away from spicy foods such as chili, pizza, hot sauce, and black pepper. Definitely avoid fatty, greasy, fried foods and fatty meats, such as hot dogs, bacon, sausages, bologna, fried chicken, fried fish, or other fried meats. Limit your intake of butter, margarine, mayonnaise, salad dressings, and other oils (fats often make diarrhea worse).

It's also a good idea to restrict your consumption of whole milk and milk products such as dips, cream sauces or soups, and whipped cream. Stick to low-fat products such as skim milk and low-fat cheese and yogurt. You might also try avoiding milk and milk products altogether for a few days to see if your diarrhea subsides. Many people cannot tolerate milk products but are able to eat low-fat yogurt and buttermilk. Speak to your nutritionist about non-dairy products if you are lactose intolerant.

Remember also to replace essential body fluids if you have diarrhea. Drink beverages such as juices, nectars, or electrolyte replacement drinks to replace vitamins and minerals your body may be losing. Try to drink eight to ten glasses of these fluids a day (at room temperature). Non-fatty soups or broths can also help replace fluids.

Avoid alcohol and caffeine, including coffee, black tea, hot chocolate, and caffeinated sodas.

Problems Chewing or Swallowing

HIV/AIDS may cause oral thrush or ulcers in the throat or mouth. This can create difficulties with chewing or swallowing. The dental problems experienced by people with HIV/AIDS can also create challenges for chewing and swallowing. Medications are available that can treat oral infections. If you're experiencing mouth sores, definitely make an appointment to speak with your dentist.

These are some guidelines for eating and drinking if you have mouth pain:

- DO puree foods in a blender if possible.
- DO cut foods into bite-sized pieces for easier chewing.
- DO add gravy, yogurt, reduced-fat mayonnaise, or evaporated skim milk to foods to make them moister.
- DO soak dry foods such as bread, crackers, cake, and cookies in milk or other beverages before eating.
- DO use a large straw for both beverages and pureed foods.
- DO eat cool foods and avoid hot foods.
- DON'T eat acidic foods such as tomato sauce, oranges, and other citrus fruits and juices if they bother you.
- DON'T eat rough foods such as raw fruits and vegetables, nuts, corn, and rice.
- DON'T consume carbonated drinks if the bubbles irritate your mouth.

Also, practice good oral hygiene. Brush with a soft-bristled toothbrush in the morning when you wake up, before you go to bed at night, and after every meal. If it isn't practical to brush after a meal, rinse your mouth with warm salt water (after snacks too). Every three months see a dentist who specializes in HIV/AIDS. You can get a referral from your doctor, your hospital, or your local AIDS service organization.

Loss of Appetite

When you feel sick, you don't feel much like eating. But, as noted earlier, it's important to maintain your weight if you have HIV/AIDS. There are ways to overcome appetite loss. Keep your portions small—a full plate can appear overwhelming. Try exercising a couple of hours before mealtime to stimulate your appetite. Avoid caffeinated drinks (including colas), which are an appetite suppressant. Keep plenty of healthy snacks handy, especially foods you like. Don't hesitate to splurge on higher price items, such as exotic fruit or gourmet crackers, if they make you want to eat. Some people have a larger appetite earlier in the day, so you may want to make your morning meal your largest. Indeed, try to get as much as one-third of your total calories at breakfast and use nutritional supplements later in the day when you don't feel like eating.

Appetite Stimulants

You can do a variety of things to make food more palatable (see above). You can also take appetite stimulants to maintain your weight and practice good nutrition. The use of "medical marijuana," an addictive substance, to increase appetite is highly controversial.

Megestrol acetate (brand name: Megace), a synthetic version of the female sex hormone progesterone, is also known to stimulate appetite. There has been some concern that Megace increases only a person's body fat; in general, however, the reported results from people who have used it have been positive. (Rarely, blood clotting occurs; Megale has also been associated with a small number of cases of breast enlargement in men.)

Vitamin and Mineral Supplements

The human body needs vitamins and minerals, or "micronutrients," to grow and rebuild cells. Healthy people can get enough vitamins and minerals from a balanced diet. Because you are sick with HIV/AIDS, you probably need more micronutrients to help repair and heal damaged cells than you can get from your diet. You also may need extra micronutrients because your medications restrict the effectiveness of the vitamins and minerals in your diet.

Unfortunately, it's not enough for people with HIV/AIDS to just take a one-a-day multivitamin to accommodate their extra needs. The amounts of vitamins and minerals in one-a-day pills are based on the Recommended Dietary

Allowances (RDAs) established by the government. However, the RDAs are the minimum amounts of micronutrients needed to prevent shortages in healthy people, not the amounts needed by someone with HIV/AIDS. Studies show that people with HIV/AIDS need between six and twenty-five times the RDAs of some vitamins and minerals.

People with HIV/AIDS will probably benefit from taking some or all of the following supplements every day at either breakfast or lunch:

- one *multivitamin supplement*
- one *beta-carotene (25,000 IU)*
- one *vitamin B-12 supplement (500 mcg)*
- one *combined calcium/magnesium/zinc (CMZ) supplement (1,000 mg/400 mg/15 mg)*
- one *iron supplement*
- one *vitamin E supplement (200 mg)*
- one *selenium supplement (400 mcg)*
- one *zinc supplement (50 mg in addition to the CMZ)*
- one *folic acid supplement*
- one *vitamin C supplement (3,000 mg)*
- one *acidophilus capsule, ten to twenty minutes after each meal*

At another meal:

- one *vitamin B-12 supplement (500 mcg)*
- one *vitamin C supplement (1,500 mg)*
- one *acidophilus capsule shortly after the meal*

Your doctor or a nutritionist who specializes in HIV/AIDS can help you design a program of supplementation that works best for you. *Remember that vitamin and mineral supplements should not be used in place of a balanced diet.*

Weight Gain Supplements

A variety of weight gain supplements are available in pharmacies and food stores. However, you should not regard weight gain supplements as a primary source of nutrition.

Protein supplements such as those used by bodybuilders are sometimes used by people with HIV/AIDS to prevent or lessen weight loss. Look for products that are high in protein and low in sugar and fat.

Weight gain protein drinks are also commonly used by people with HIV/AIDS. To get the most benefit from protein drinks, use them in conjunction with exercise.

Food and Water Safety

If you have HIV/AIDS, what you put in your body is very important. Even minor contaminations can cause major problems.

Food

It is extremely important to avoid the potential for bacterial and parasitic contamination when preparing food. Your compromised immune system will make it very difficult for you to fight an infection caused by such contamination. These are some simple guidelines to help you keep your meals free of harmful contaminants:

- Wash fruits and vegetables thoroughly, as this can remove many organisms found in soil. Use a vegetable brush to remove soil and chemical residues.
- Avoid eating fresh vegetables and salads at restaurants or anywhere else where you can't be certain that the products were washed adequately.
- Avoid eating raw eggs and food containing raw eggs. In recent years there have been thousands of cases of salmonella poisoning from Caesar salad dressing made with raw eggs. If you choose to eat salads at restaurants (despite these

guidelines), be sure to ask whether raw eggs are used in salad dressings and other foods.

- Cook meat thoroughly, at least 140 degrees Fahrenheit. Avoid "pink" meat, including rare steaks and burgers and uncooked meat or fish, including sushi. Bacterias that cause diseases such as salmonellosis and toxoplasmosis, as well as parasites, are found in raw and under-cooked chicken, beef, pork, and fish.
- Use different cutting boards for foods that will be cooked and for those served raw. For example, salads that are prepared on a cutting board that has just been used for preparing meat can become contaminated by organisms in the meat.
- Wash hands, kitchen utensils, and cutting boards frequently and thoroughly during food preparation. Avoid allowing meat juices to contaminate cheese, vegetables, and other foods.
- Keep kitchen appliances, shelves, countertops, refrigerators, freezers, and utensils clean, and wash sponges and towels frequently. To kill germs, heat sponges in the microwave for one minute or put them in the dishwasher.
- Wash all utensils and your hands with soap and water between handling one food and handling another in order to help prevent cross-contamination.

- Thaw meats in the refrigerator rather than in the open air, keeping the refrigerator temperature at 40 degrees Fahrenheit or lower.

Water

It's also important to pay attention to the safety of the water you drink. Cryptosporidiosis, or "crypto" as it's usually called, is the most serious illness caused by drinking contaminated water, and cryptosporidia are found in the water systems of many communities. Crypto is among the most common causes of diarrhea in people in the United States with HIV/AIDS. Assume all tap water contains cryptosporidia. The easiest way to find out if your municipal water system contains cryptosporidia is to call your local water utility and ask about the source of your drinking water, whether it is susceptible to contaminants, and how the water is treated and tested.

These are some safe drinking water sources:

- tap water that has been at a full and rolling boil for one minute.
- bottled water that is certified free of parasites or that has been subjected to one of the following: distillation, reverse osmosis, or absolute one-micron filtration. For information, call your local

bottler or the International Bottled Water Association (IBWA) at (800) WATER-11 (928-3711).
- point-of-use filters for the faucet that are certified NSF 53 for cyst removal. Be aware that filter cartridges are expensive and must frequently be changed. Whenever you change a filter, wear rubber gloves since all the contaminants that the filter took out of the water are now in the cartridge. If you don't wear gloves, these contaminants may get on your hands and eventually wind up in your stomach. Of course, wash the gloves in warm soapy water or throw them away after use. When you are finished, wash your hands with warm soapy water for twenty seconds.

If you think you have been infected with crypto, see your doctor immediately. Routine stool tests used for most parasites do not detect cryptosporidium. Therefore, you will need a special test to find out if you have crypto.

Exercise

Physical exercise improves health and is an effective supportive HIV/AIDS treatment. The two main forms of physical exercise that benefit people with HIV/AIDS are aerobic exercise and resistance training.

Aerobic Exercise

Aerobic exercise gets the heart and lungs working faster and therefore makes them stronger. For people with HIV who are symptom-free, vigorous regular aerobic exercise (sometimes called "cardiovascular" exercise), lasting thirty to forty-five minutes, three to four times per week, provides a solid heart-lung workout. Examples of aerobic exercise include running, biking, dancing, aerobics classes, swimming, cross-country skiing, roller-blading, games such as soccer, racquetball, and basketball, and use of cardiovascular machines such as stair climbers, stationary bikes, and treadmills. Many people cross-train—participate in a variety of forms of exercise—to keep up their interest and motivation.

In addition to strengthening the heart and lungs, an aerobic exercise program combats depression by raising endorphin levels. In several studies, aerobic exercise actually raised CD4+ counts (an indicator of the strength of the immune system). One study showed fewer opportunistic infections and better stress-coping skills in a group of regular exercisers. Marathons and other extreme endurance workouts, however, can weaken the immune system.

Resistance Training

Resistance training uses weights or machines to build muscle mass and help preserve lean body weight. Losing muscle mass, known as "wasting," is a key problem for HIV-positive men and women. A program of resistance training can be done by lifting weights (barbells, dumbbells, and weight machines) or by using your own weight as the resistance (push-ups and sit-ups). Strength training is a safe and effective way to increase muscle mass, reduce fat, and maintain or increase a healthy weight. Doctors are developing a strength-training regimen especially for people with HIV/AIDS. In the meantime, ask your doctor if you can follow general guidelines for strength training:

- Work out at least two times but not more than three times per week. If you are not interested in large strength gains, you can get almost as much improvement (70 to 80 percent as much) by doing strength training two times a week instead of three.
- Include eight to ten exercises that use major muscle groups in both the upper and lower body (arms, shoulders, chest, abdomen, back, hips, and legs).

- Do at least one set of each exercise, and no more than three.
- Each set should consist of ten to fifteen repetitions, which should nearly exhaust the muscle group being exercised.
- Make your strength-training session last between twenty and fifty minutes.
- Do the exercise through the full range of movement, and don't jerk or overly strain to lift the weight.

If you are symptomatic or recovering from illness, it's important to discuss a specific exercise program with your health care provider. Physical therapists are trained to help develop rehabilitation programs. Regardless of your health status, always begin exercise gently and build slowly. In almost all cases, any exercise is better than none at all.

Benefits of Exercise

Aerobic Exercise

- *reduces the risk of heart disease, stroke, and high blood pressure by strengthening the heart and lungs*
- *combats depression by raising endorphin levels*

- *lowers the risk of opportunistic infections in people with HIV/AIDS*
- *done in a health-club-type environment, provides a positive social environment*

Resistance Exercise

- *counteracts the risk of "wasting" (loss of muscle mass)*
- *combats depression by raising endorphin levels*
- *done in a health-club-type environment, provides a positive social environment*

A Beginner's Walking Program

The beginner's walking program is designed for people who haven't exercised for some time. Even if you are very unfit, you can do the walking sessions described in the early part of the program. Each walking session is divided into three parts: the warm-up phase, the target zone phase, and the cool-down phase. Of these three phases, the target zone requires explanation.

Achieving the Target Zone

To get the maximum benefit from exercise, it is necessary to exercise hard enough that your heart and lungs are working at between 60 and 75 percent of their maximum capabilities.

To see if your heart rate is within your target zone, you need to check your pulse while you're exercising. Here's how:

- Place the tips of your fingers over one of the major blood vessels (try just to the left or right of your Adam's apple or the spot on the inside of your wrist below the bone of your thumb).
- Count the number of times your heart beats during a ten-second period. Then multiply that number by six to figure out how many times a minute your heart is beating.
- Compare your heart rate with the following chart. For instance, if you are sixty-five years old, your goal is to have a target zone of between 78 and 116 beats per minute.

Age	Target Heart Rate Zone
20 years	100–150 beats per minute
25 years	98–146 beats per minute
30 years	95–142 beats per minute
35 years	93–138 beats per minute
40 years	90–135 beats per minute

Age	Target Heart Rate Zone
45 years	88–131 beats per minute
50 years	85–127 beats per minute
55 years	83–123 beats per minute
60 years	80–120 beats per minute
65 years	78–116 beats per minute
70 years	75–113 beats per minute

Each week do the walking session three times, as shown for week 1. If you find you reach a point where the sessions leave you overly fatigued (tired enough that you don't think you could go to the next level), repeat that week's program until you think you are fit enough to move on to the next level. You don't have to complete the program in twelve weeks.

	Warm-Up Phase	Target Zone Phase	Cool-Down Phase	Total
Week 1				
Session A	Walk normally, 5 min.	Walk fast, 5 min.	Walk normally, 5 min.	15 min.
Session B	repeat	repeat	repeat	repeat
Session C	repeat	repeat	repeat	repeat

	Warm-Up Phase	Target Zone Phase	Cool-Down Phase	Total
Week 2	Walk normally, 5 min.	Walk fast, 7 min.	Walk normally, 5 min.	17 min.
Week 3	Walk normally, 5 min.	Walk fast, 9 min.	Walk normally, 5 min.	19 min.
Week 4	Walk normally, 5 min.	Walk fast, 11 min.	Walk normally, 5 min.	21 min.
Week 5	Walk normally, 5 min.	Walk fast, 13 min.	Walk normally, 5 min.	23 min.
Week 6	Walk normally, 5 min.	Walk fast, 15 min.	Walk normally, 5 min.	25 min.
Week 7	Walk normally, 5 min.	Walk fast, 18 min.	Walk normally, 5 min.	28 min.
Week 8	Walk normally, 5 min.	Walk fast, 20 min.	Walk normally, 5 min.	30 min.
Week 9	Walk normally, 5 min.	Walk fast, 23 min.	Walk normally, 5 min.	33 min.
Week 10	Walk normally, 5 min.	Walk fast, 26 min.	Walk normally, 5 min.	36 min.

	Warm-Up Phase	Target Zone Phase	Cool-Down Phase	Total
Week 11	Walk normally, 5 min.	Walk fast, 28 min.	Walk normally, 5 min.	38 min.
Week 12	Walk normally, 5 min.	Walk fast, 30 min.	Walk normally, 5 min.	40 min.

Week 13 onward: Remember to check your pulse periodically during the target zone phase to make sure you are exercising in that zone. As your lungs adapt to the demands of this walking program, try exercising in the upper range of your target zone. Gradually increase your fast-walking time to between thirty and sixty minutes three or four times a week. With a five-minute warm-up and cool-down period, your walking sessions should last from forty to seventy minutes.

CHAPTER SIX

Women and HIV/AIDS

More women in the United States are being infected with HIV and getting AIDS. In 1995, only 7 percent of AIDS cases were women, but by 1997, that figure was 20 percent. An estimated 107,000 to 150,000 women in the United States are HIV-positive. Many of these women have not developed AIDS. Minority women in the United States are disproportionately affected by AIDS. In 1996, 56 percent of reported female AIDS cases in the United States were African American women and 20 percent were Hispanic women. HIV infection is presently the third-leading cause of death in women in the twenty-five to forty-four age group and is the leading cause of death in black women of that age group. Worldwide, almost half of the adults living with HIV/AIDS are women.

Like men, women with HIV/AIDS are susceptible to conditions such as Pneumocystis carinii pneumonia (PCP), but they also suffer gender-specific illnesses such as recurrent vaginal yeast infections and pelvic inflammatory disease (PID).

Women who are HIV-positive often have difficulty getting health care. Frequently they are preoccupied with caring for other family members, especially children. In addition, they may lack support and face other challenges that interfere with treatment therapies.

Much more study needs to be done on HIV infection in pregnant and nonpregnant women: how it is transmitted, how it progresses, and the symptoms. Researchers are studying the unique aspects of HIV/AIDS in women and developing new treatments for infected women.

Scientists are also working on new methods of HIV prevention. These include creams and gels that women can apply before sex to protect against HIV and other sexually transmitted diseases (STDs). Many of these studies are being conducted by the National Institute of Allergy and Infectious Diseases (NIAID), which is part of the National Institutes of Health.

Another important area of research is mother-to-child transmission. Researchers are investigating ways to reduce such occurrences. For instance, a specific regimen of zidovudine (AZT), given to an HIV-infected woman during pregnancy and to her infant after birth, appears to reduce mother-to-baby transmission by two-thirds. Other drug regimens are also being developed that may be even more effective, as well as simpler and less costly.

How HIV Is Transmitted to Women

Among U.S. women, the HIV infection is most commonly transmitted during sex with an HIV-positive man or while using HIV-contaminated syringes to inject narcotics such as heroin, cocaine, or amphetamines. In the United States in 1996, 66 percent of AIDS cases among women were attributed to heterosexual contact and 34 percent to injection drug use.

Women are more vulnerable than men to being infected with HIV during heterosexual sex. Studies show that a woman who has other sexually transmitted diseases—particularly infections that cause ulcerations of the mucosal surfaces (such as syphilis and chancroid)—has a much greater risk of getting infected with HIV. Anal sex also increases the risk a woman will become infected with HIV.

Other factors thought to increase the likelihood of HIV transmission through heterosexual sex include alcohol use, history of childhood sexual abuse, current domestic abuse, and use of crack cocaine.

Using condoms reduces the risk of HIV transmission. In studies of heterosexual couples wherein one is HIV-positive and the other is not, use of condoms kept transmission rates extremely low.

Signs and Symptoms

HIV affects men and women in many of the same ways. Males and females infected with HIV may have vague symptoms even early in the progression of the disease, including low-grade fevers, night sweats, fatigue, and weight loss. In the United States, the most common AIDS-related condition in both men and women is Pneumocystis carinii pneumonia (PCP). Therapies to fight the virus, and those used to treat opportunistic infections, are as effective in women as in men.

Other conditions occur in different frequencies in men and women. HIV-infected men, for instance, are eight times more likely than women to develop Kaposi's sarcoma. Certain studies have shown that women have higher rates of esophageal candidiasis (yeast infections of the trachea or windpipe) and herpes simplex infections than men. Women have also been found to suffer more often from bacterial pneumonia, though this has been attributed to factors such as a delay in seeking care among HIV-positive women as compared with men and/or less access to treatment and prevention.

Female-Specific Symptoms

Women with HIV also experience gynecological problems associated with their HIV. Most of these problems also occur in women who do not have HIV but less often and not as severely.

Vaginal yeast infections, which are common in women and easily treated, occur more frequently in HIV-positive women and are harder to treat. A drug called fluconazole is often used to treat yeast infections. Weekly doses of fluconazole can also safely *prevent* vaginal and esophageal candidiasis without causing unwanted resistance to the drug.

Bacterial vaginosis and common STDs such as *gonorrhea, chlamydia,* and *trichomoniasis* are other vaginal infections that may occur more often and be more severe in HIV-infected women.

Severe *herpes simplex* outbreaks, sometimes unresponsive to the standard drug used to treat the condition, can severely affect a woman's quality of life.

Genital ulcers are a unique consequence of HIV. These ulcers, for which there is no cure or treatment, are sometimes confused with breakouts of herpes simplex. Studies are under way to determine whether thalidomide may be an effective treatment for this condition.

Human papillomavirus (HPV) infections, which cause genital warts and can lead to cervical cancer, occur with disproportionate frequency in HIV-positive women. A precancerous condition associated with HPV called *cervical intraepithelial neoplasia*

(CIN) also is more common and severe in women infected with HIV and more likely to recur after treatment. Several studies are under way to test different treatments for CIN.

Pelvic inflammatory disease (PID) seems to be more prevalent and aggressive in HIV-infected women than in women who do not have the disease. PID may become a chronic and relapsing condition as a woman's immune system deteriorates.

The Need for Gynecological Screening

HIV-positive women should have a complete gynecological evaluation, including a Pap smear, as part of their initial HIV evaluation or upon beginning prenatal care and another Pap smear six months later. If both smears are negative, annual screening should be done in women with no HIV symptoms. More frequent screening every six months is recommended for HIV-positive women who are experiencing HIV symptoms or signs of human papillomavirus infection or who have had prior abnormal Pap smears.

Importance of Early Diagnosis

Particular groups of American women have limited access to proper health care. In addition, many women do not believe they are at risk of being infected with HIV. For these and other reasons, symptoms that should be warnings for HIV infection, such as recurrent yeast infections, often go unheeded. PID, chronic interstitial nephritis, and the female-specific symptoms described on pages 132–134 should immediately prompt health care workers to offer women HIV testing as well as counseling.

Early diagnosis of HIV enables women to get a head start on antiviral medications and drugs to prevent opportunistic infections, both of which can delay the development of AIDS and, in so doing, prolong life. Early diagnosis also enables women to make informed choices about conception and pregnancy. Health care workers should be alert to early signs of HIV infection in women, and all women who have engaged in high-risk activities should be tested (see page 9 for information on who should be tested).

Survival Times in HIV-Positive Women

When HIV infection is detected and treatment begins right away, a woman's survival time is the same as that for a man. Women, however, are less likely than men to get early diagnosis and treatment, so in reality survival times in women are shorter than in men.

In one study of more than 4,500 men and women with HIV, the women were one-third more likely than the men to die within the study period. The researchers could not determine precisely the reasons for the higher mortality rate in the women participants but speculated that poorer access to or use of health care resources among HIV-infected women was one probable cause. Other contributory factors included homelessness and lack of social support for women.

Mother-to-Child Transmission of HIV

HIV can be transmitted from mother to child in the following ways:

- through pregnancy
- during labor and delivery
- through breast feeding

In the United States, approximately 25 percent of pregnant HIV-positive women not receiving AZT have transmitted the virus to their babies. Most prenatal infections—an estimated 50 to 80 percent—probably occur late in pregnancy or during birth. Although exactly how HIV is passed from mother to child is unknown, researchers think the virus may be transmitted when the mother's blood enters the fetal circulation or by mucosal exposure to the virus during labor and delivery. Researchers are unclear as to the role of the placenta and are studying this aspect of perinatal transmission.

The risk of mother-to-child transmission is greatly

increased if the mother has advanced HIV disease, large amounts of the virus in her bloodstream, or only small amounts of CD4+ cells.

Other factors that may increase the risk of mother-to-child transmission are drug use by the mother, severe inflammation of the fetal membrane, or a prolonged period between fetal membrane rupture and delivery. A recent study showed that HIV-infected women who gave birth more than four hours after the rupture of the fetal membrane were almost twice as likely to transmit HIV to their infants, versus those who delivered in less than four hours after fetal membrane rupture. The same study showed that HIV-positive women who used heroin or crack cocaine during their pregnancies were almost twice as likely to transmit HIV to their children compared with HIV-positive women who had not abused these substances.

HIV is also transmitted from a nursing mother to her infant. A recent study showed that women with HIV who breast-feed have a 10 percent chance of passing on the virus to their infants.

CHAPTER SEVEN

Complementary and Alternative Treatments for HIV/AIDS

You have turned over control of your disease to a Higher Power. In doing so, you have agreed to do your part in taking care of yourself. That includes finding out what treatments are available that may help alleviate or improve your condition, even those treatments outside the realm of "conventional" medicine.

Complementary and alternative medicines are treatments and health care approaches not taught widely in Western medical schools, not generally used in hospitals, and not usually reimbursed by medical insurance. The terms cover a wide range of ancient healing philosophies, approaches, and therapies.

The terms "alternative" and "complementary" are not interchangeable. Therapies used *instead of* conventional medicine are considered to be alternative. Therapies used *in conjunction with* conventional medicine are referred to as complementary.

Certain complementary and alternative approaches are based on familiar principles of Western medicine, but many have quite different origins. Many therapies remain far outside the realm of accepted Western medicine, while others have been embraced by large segments of society.

Consider, for instance, the ancient Chinese medical practice of acupuncture. Once considered quite bizarre in the West, acupuncture is now increasingly used by ordinary Americans to treat common medical conditions, to relieve stress, and even to ease symptoms during nicotine withdrawal. The same is true for herbal medicine, as evidenced by the television commercials for products containing echinacea, ginseng, and Saint-John's-wort. Given their increasing popularity among those attracted by low cost, lack of side effects, and purported effectiveness, many forms of medicine presently considered "offbeat" will eventually become accepted by mainstream health culture.

Society's interest in alternatives to conventional medicine led the government-run National Institutes of Health (NIH) to create an Office of Alternative Medicine (OAM) in 1992. The OAM facilitates research and evaluation of unconventional medical practices and disseminates this information to the public. Its budget in 1998 was $20 million. You can obtain a classification of forty-seven complementary and alternative medical health care practices from the OAM. The list is intended to show the diversity of the field and is neither complete nor authoritative.

Many practitioners of conventional health care continue to dispute the claims of alternative and complementary medicine because, by and large, such therapies are not investigated using the same scientific research methods used in conventional medicine. The benefits of such treatments, Western-trained doctors argue, are strictly "anecdotal," that is, based on patient testimonials, not on documented results. It is unlikely that alternative and complementary medicine will be fully accepted until its practitioners can produce results based on rigorous research methods, which in turn depend on systematic, explicit, and comprehensive knowledge and skills.

Finding Out More about Complementary and Alternative Treatments for HIV/AIDS

Health care providers are becoming more familiar with alternative and complementary treatments, and your doctor may be willing to refer you to such a practitioner. The medical profession, however, is by and large suspicious of medical treatments it considers untested and unproved, and thus potentially harmful.

Don't be discouraged if your doctor cannot or will not provide you with the information you want. Good sources of information about particular complementary and alternative medical practices are available on the Internet, in medical libraries, in public libraries, and in popular bookstores.

Other resources for alternative and complementary therapies are the NIH's twenty-four institutes, centers, and divisions. For information from the NIH on HIV/AIDS, call (301) 496-4000 and ask the operator to direct you to the appropriate office.

An excellent online source of complementary and alternative medicine is the alternative medicine section of www.healthanswers.com.

A growing number of professional associations, educational organizations, and research institutions provide information about complementary and alternative medical practices. Many of these organizations have sites on the Internet.

Be aware that some of these organizations advocate a specific therapy or treatment but are unable to provide complete and objective health information. Before trying out any treatment, make sure to get as much information as you can and to discuss your findings and thoughts with your doctor.

How to Find a Practitioner in Your Area

To find a qualified complementary and/or alternative medical health care practitioner, contact medical regulatory and licensing agencies in your state (your health care provider should be able to provide you with their names). Such regulatory and licensing bodies can provide information about a specific practitioner's credentials and background. Many states license practitioners who provide alternative therapies such as acupuncture, chiropractic services, and massage therapy.

You may also locate individual practitioners by asking your health care provider or by contacting a professional association or organization. These organizations can provide names of local practitioners and information about how to determine the quality of a specific practitioner's services.

Choosing an Alternative Health Care Therapy or Practitioner

The health decisions you make are important, and choosing to explore complementary and alternative treatments is no exception. There are some serious issues you need to address when selecting an alternative or a complementary therapy or practitioner. In particular, ask yourself questions about the safety and effectiveness of the treatment, the qualifications of the practitioner, and the cost of the therapy.

Is It Safe? Is It Effective?

The therapy should provide relief from the condition for which it is sought—in this case, HIV/AIDS—and it should not have the ability to cause you harm when used as intended. Unfortunately, less is known about the safety and effectiveness of complementary and alternative products and practices than conventional medicine. So what can you do?

Ask the alternative/complementary health practitioner for evidence of the safety and effectiveness of the practice, treatment, or technology he or she advocates. Request information on new research that either supports or debunks the effectiveness of the treatment, and also ask about any new information concerning its safety.

You should also ask questions about possible side effects, interactions with other medications you are taking, expected results, and how long the treatment should last.

Make sure the practitioner is aware of all other therapies—both conventional and alternative/ complementary—you are using, as this information will probably be necessary to ensure the safety and effectiveness of the treatment plan.

Published information on the safety and effectiveness of particular therapies can be found in scientific
journals available at certain public libraries, university libraries, medical libraries, online computer services, and the U.S. National Library of Medicine
(NLM) at the National Institutes of Health. As the articles in these journals can be difficult for the lay-
person to understand, you might find the summary at
the beginning of the manuscript, known as the "ab-
stract," the easiest way to gain information from these
materials. You can find these scientific articles in the
Index Medicus, a published resource available in medical and university libraries and some public libraries.

The World Wide Web can be an excellent source of
information about the safety and effectiveness of
complementary and alternative medicine, although it
is important that you learn to differentiate between
credible and noncredible sources. This ability to dis-
cern comes in part with time spent using the Internet.

Also try to gain access to people with HIV/AIDS
who have received the treatment you are researching.
Remember, though, that anecdotal evidence from
other patients is not an accurate measure of the safety
and effectiveness of a treatment. Therefore, it should
not be the sole criterion for selecting an alternative
or a complementary therapy. Studies done under

controlled conditions by trained medical scientists
are the best way to assess a treatment's effectiveness.

What Are the Practitioner's Qualifications?

Research the background, qualifications, and reputation of the practitioner. You can do this by contacting
the state or local regulatory body that has jurisdic-
tion over the practice of the therapy you are seeking.
Although complementary and alternative medicine
is not as strictly regulated as conventional medicine,
licensing and accreditation are continually being
introduced.

Local and state medical boards may be able to provide information about an individual practitioner's
credentials, and consumer affairs departments such as
the Better Business Bureau can tell you whether any
complaints have been lodged against that person.

How Much Does It Cost?

Your health insurer or the practitioner should be able
to tell you whether a particular therapy is covered by
insurance. However, most complementary and alternative treatments are not covered by health insurance. Patients usually have to pay the entire amount
of the therapy. Thus cost is a very important factor
for people seeking alternative and complementary
medical treatment.

"Shop around" to find out what different practitioners charge for the same service. Although cost shouldn't be the sole criterion for selection, knowing what a variety of practitioners charge will give you some idea of what is appropriate. The same professional and regulatory bodies that can provide information on safety and effectiveness should be able to provide approximate cost guidelines.

Specific Alternative/Complementary Treatments for HIV/AIDS

Studies indicate that from 25 to 75 percent of people with HIV/AIDS have tried some form of alternative or complementary medicine. The following sections contain information on treatments that may be considered in creating a comprehensive, holistic, and assertive approach to treating HIV/AIDS. No endorsement of any particular approach is intended or should be inferred.

Acupuncture and Chinese Herbs

More than 20 percent of the planet's population uses Chinese medicine—an ancient form of treatments that emphasize treating the whole person, not just a particular disease. In other words, two people with HIV/AIDS may be treated very differently using

Chinese medicine, depending on their strengths, weaknesses, imbalances, and general lifestyle.

Despite this emphasis on individualized treatments, standard herbal and acupuncture protocols have been developed for treating HIV. Several studies show that formulas with astragalus, lingustrum, ginseng, licorice, and other Chinese herbs are effective against symptoms such as fatigue, night sweats, weight loss, diarrhea, and skin rashes. These herbs have not been shown to decrease amounts of the AIDS virus in a patient's body.

A common practice among HIV/AIDS patients is to add one of the standard astragalus-based herbal formulas to their conventional drug treatment regimen. If you want to explore the use of Chinese herbalism further, seek the counsel of a practitioner of Chinese medicine experienced in treating people with HIV. Various ways exist to incorporate Chinese medicine into conventional treatments for HIV/AIDS. In fact, one of the strengths of Chinese medicine is its ability to relieve the side effects of standard prescription drugs.

Herbs and Natural Medicines

From the beginning of the HIV/AIDS pandemic when no approved drugs existed, people with HIV/AIDS were attracted to herbal and nonsynthetic alternatives. Some of these had a reputation for boosting the immune system, while others were reputed to work against viruses; several were specifically intended for use against HIV/AIDS. Early on the recommendations for use were based on folklore and anecdotal information. Now a few of these medicines have been tested in clinical trials. *Natural doesn't always mean safe*—especially for people with HIV/AIDS. The risks and benefits of any HIV/AIDS treatment must be weighed.

The following are among the herbal and natural remedies used by people with HIV/AIDS.

Compound Q

Derived from the root of the Chinese cucumber, this medicine is sold through buyers' clubs for HIV/AIDS and is given intravenously. Only doctors willing to work with unapproved products or at "underground" clinics will prescribe it. Unlike most other antivirals, which slow the spread of the virus to uninfected cells, Compound Q kills already infected cells. Results in certain cases have been very impressive, increasing CD4+ counts dramatically, but more often, stabilizing these counts that would otherwise continue declining. There is a wide variety in dosages being used, frequency of administering the dosages, and the duration of the infusion. Side effects such as muscle aches and fatigue can be minimized by over-the-counter pain medications such as ibuprofen. In rare cases, a life-threatening allergic reaction known as anaphylaxis has occurred. Other serious side effects have been seen in people with low CD4+ counts. These may be prevented with pretreatments of Decadron and by screening out people with low CD4+ counts. Anyone with CD4+ counts under 100 should approach using Compound Q with great caution, if not avoid using it altogether. Whenever it is used, this medicine must be prescribed and administered by someone experienced with it and prepared for the emergency treatment of anaphylaxis.

Hypericin

Hypericin, an extract from the flower of Saint-John's-wort, has been shown in certain studies to have an antiviral effect against HIV by stopping the virus from replicating. However, initial intravenous administration of completely natural concentrations of the drug resulted in severe side effects. Synthetic versions in oral form produce less intense side effects, though studies have been sparse.

Echinacea and Other Immune System Stimulants

Several natural substances stimulate the immune system. These include echinacea, mistletoe (*Viscum album*), goldenseal, shiitake mushrooms, aloe (acemannen), and garlic. Although these substances have been shown to stimulate the immune system, how to harness their powers so they benefit people with HIV is not so well known. And just because something is known to boost the immune system does not mean it is necessarily beneficial; boosting certain parts of the immune system can compromise others, leading to virus progression. Furthermore, using excess amounts of substances such as garlic or mushrooms can upset the body's balance of antibiotics and fungi and interfere with the effectiveness of standard treatments for HIV. Clinical trials are currently being conducted to test how best to use some of these substances to treat people with HIV/AIDS.

Curmucin

One of the elements of the herb turmeric, curmucin has been shown to slow HIV replication in test tubes. Although tests are still being done, the attractiveness of this substance is considerable because it is so inexpensive and widely available.

Shark Cartilage

The cartilage of sharks contains natural antibiotics and other substances that may slow the progression of HIV. Because shark cartilage smells so unpleasant and tends to cause nausea and stomach upset, it is usually administered as a retention enema. Tested on only a small number of people, shark cartilage has proven effective in some cases.

Kombucha

A living, growing colony of fungal and bacterial elements also known as the Manchurian mushroom, kombucha is brewed and taken as a tea for its purported immune-enhancing and antibiotic properties. There have been several well-publicized reports of increases in CD4+ counts, and frequent reports of increased energy and alertness. Concern has been raised that other disease-causing germs might also be growing in this substance and that, because of its antibiotic properties, resistance might develop toward certain diseases. In particular, people with low CD4+ counts should be wary of taking this treatment.

Ozone

Ozone, an unstable form of oxygen, is used commercially to kill bacteria. The theory is that because high oxygen levels kill many microbes, then ozone will kill HIV. In people with HIV/AIDS, ozone is administered in a variety of ways—intravenously, rectally, and ex-vivo infusion (blood is drawn, mixed with ozone, then put back in the body). Although this therapy has many proponents, and many people with HIV/AIDS have sought it out, the fact is that only 1 percent of the HIV in a person's body is in the blood itself—most of it lives in other parts of the body, including the lymph nodes, cells, and other organs. There is little evidence to support this therapy.

Hyperthermia

Many proponents of natural healing believe that fever is the body's way to combat infection. By extension, heating the blood will help fight HIV, they believe. However, after several reports released in the 1980s stated that hyperthermia was not beneficial, the treatment was banned in the United States. Several Americans have died as a result of receiving this treatment abroad. The major objection to hyperthermia is the same as it is for ozone—that is, little HIV is actually in the blood. Most of the virus is in other parts of the body where hyperthermia will have little effect.

Homeopathy

Homeopathy is an immensely popular approach to healing in Europe and has developed a following in the United States too. People with HIV/AIDS are drawn to homeopathy because it is nontoxic. Unlike conventional Western medicine, which attacks disease head-on with medicines such as antibiotics, homeopathic medicine treats "like with like." Homeopathy practitioners use substances that actually cause the symptoms of the disease to be treated. When administered in dilute form, these substances are believed to cure the disease that causes the symptoms.

Many people with HIV/AIDS have reported significant reduction in their symptoms using homeopathic remedies. Recent research has begun to challenge the medical establishment's bias against this centuries-old medical approach.

Alternative or complementary treatments should not be a substitute for any HIV/AIDS treatments prescribed by your doctor. Before you use an alternative or a complementary treatment, carefully discuss this decision with your doctor.

Appendix

National AIDS Hotlines and Resources

The following organizations provide extensive information about HIV/AIDS. Consider volunteering at one of these organizations.

The Americans with Disabilities Act Information and Assistance Hotline: (800) 949-4232 V/TTY

The Centers for Disease Control (CDC)
National AIDS Hotline: (800) 342-AIDS (800-342-2437) (twenty-four hours a day, daily) TTY/TDD: (800) AIDS-TTY (800-243-7889)
English Hotline: (800) 342-AIDS (800-342-2437)
Spanish Hotline: (800) 344-SIDA (800-344-7432)

The Centers for Disease Control (CDC)
National AIDS Prevention Information Network: (800) 458-5231 (Monday–Friday, 9:00 A.M.–6:00 P.M., eastern time) TTY/TDD: (800) 243-7012
International Line: (301) 562-1098

Providing free educational materials about HIV and
other sexually transmitted diseases.

The Centers for Disease Control (CDC)
National Sexually Transmitted Diseases Hotline:
(800) 227-8922 (Monday–Friday, 8:00 A.M.–11:00
P.M., eastern time)
Anonymous, confidential information about sexually
transmitted diseases and how to prevent them. Also
provides referrals to clinical and other services.

The Gay and Lesbian National Hotline:
(888) THE-GLNH (888-843-4564) Monday–Friday,
6:00 P.M.–10:00 P.M.; Saturday, 12:00 P.M.–5:00 P.M.,
eastern time)
A nonprofit organization providing nationwide toll-
free counseling, information, and referrals.

Hemophilia AIDS Network/National Hemophilia
Foundation: (800) 424-2634

National Association of People with AIDS:
(202) 898-0414 Hotline and TTY/TDD

National Herpes Hotline: (919) 361-8488

National Pediatric/Family HIV Resource Center:
(800) 362-0071

Women Alive: (800) 554-4876 (Monday,
Wednesday, Friday, 11:00 A.M.–6:00 P.M.,
Pacific time)
A national hotline staffed by HIV-positive women
volunteers. Aimed at HIV-positive women who need
peer support or treatment information. Spanish-
speaking operators are available.

Treatment Hotlines

AIDS Clinical Trials Information Service (ACTIS):
(800) TRIALS-A (800-874-2572)
HIV/AIDS Treatment Information Service (ATIS):
(800) HIV-0440 (800-448-0440) or (301) 519-0459
Hearing-impaired access: (800) 243-7012
(Monday–Friday, 9:00 A.M.–7:00 P.M. eastern time)
Callers can speak with experienced health special-
ists for help in locating HIV/AIDS clinical trials
across the United States. Spanish-speaking special-
ists are available.

AIDS Treatment Data Network: (800) 734-7104
or (212) 260-8868 (Spanish-speaking operators
available.)

Project Inform
National HIV Treatment Line: (800) 822-7422
(Monday–Friday, 9:00 A.M.–5:00 P.M.; Saturday,
10:00 A.M.–4:00 P.M., Pacific time)
International Hotline: (415) 558-9051

Index

A

abacavir, 64, 66, 72

acceptance, ix, x, 20, 21
  of HIV diagnosis, xxii, 17, 22
  of self, 28, 29, 31, 34, 41

acemannen, 149–50

acquired immune deficiency syndrome. *See* AIDS

acupuncture, 140, 148

addictions, ix, xiii, 20, 60–62

aerobic exercise, 120, 122–23

African American women, 129

Agenerase, 65, 68

AIDS, 2–3
  alternative/complementary medicine for, 147–54
  deaths from, 1, 129

psychological impact of, 18, 83–86
  symptoms of, 7–8
  See also HIV

AIDS Clinical Trials Information Services (ACTIS), 16, 81, 157

Alcoholics Anonymous, ix, xi, xii, xxi, 60, 89
  Promises of, xiii, xxi–xxii

Alcoholics Anonymous World Services, 88

alcohol use, 60, 61, 62, 131

Aldesleukin, 76

aloe, 149–50

alternative treatments, 53, 139–47
  acceptance of, 140, 141
  for HIV/AIDS, 147–54
  insurance coverage for, 139, 146
  practitioners of, 143–44, 146–47

About the Author

MARK JENKINS is the author of several books on health. He co-wrote *The Sports Medicine Bible,* a Book-of-the-Month Club alternate selection. Jenkins lives year-round on the island of Martha's Vineyard off the coast of Cape Cod, Massachusetts. He travels occasionally to the mainland by ferryboat to fulfill his duties as publishing consultant at the world-renowned Boston Children's Hospital.

HAZELDEN INFORMATION AND EDUCATIONAL SERVICES is a division of the Hazelden Foundation, a not-for-profit organization. Since 1949, Hazelden has been a leader in promoting the dignity and treatment of people afflicted with the disease of chemical dependency.

The mission of the foundation is to improve the quality of life for individuals, families, and communities by providing a national continuum of information, education, and recovery services that are widely accessible; to advance the field through research and training; and to improve our quality and effectiveness through continuous improvement and innovation.

Stemming from that, the mission of this division is to provide quality information and support to people wherever they may be in their personal journey—from education and early intervention, through treatment and recovery, to personal and spiritual growth.

Although our treatment programs do not necessarily use everything Hazelden publishes, our bibliotherapeutic materials support our mission and the Twelve Step philosophy upon which it is based. We encourage your comments and feedback.

The headquarters of the Hazelden Foundation is in Center City, Minnesota. Additional treatment facilities are located in Chicago, Illinois; New York, New York; Plymouth, Minnesota; St. Paul, Minnesota; and West Palm Beach, Florida. At these sites, we provide a continuum of care for men and women of all ages. Our Plymouth facility is designed specifically for youth and families.

For more information on Hazelden, please call **1-800-257-7800.** Or you may access our World Wide Web site on the Internet at **www.hazelden.org.**